Working and Learning

Working and Learning

The Learning Environment in Clinical Nursing

Margaret E Ogier

SRN SCM DipN RNT BSc(Hons) PhD(Lond) C Psychol

Scutari Press
London

A division of Scutari Projects, the publishing
company of the Royal College of Nursing

First published 1989

British Library Cataloguing in Publication Data

Ogier, Margaret E.
  Working and learning : the learning environment in
  clinical nursing.
  1. Medicine. Nursing
  I. Title
  610.73

  ISBN 1 871364 23 X

Typeset by Photo·graphics
Printed and bound in Great Britain by Billing & Sons, Worcester

Contents

Preface

Working and Learning is aimed at the clinical nurse, ward sister, head nurse, supervisor and staff nurse, whether she works in a hospital ward, department or clinic, or in the community. The purpose of the book is to help the clinical nurse raise her awareness of her own need, and that of her colleagues and subordinates, to be constantly updating her current knowledge, skills and attitudes, as well as to increase a desire for professional development and personal growth.

By considering some current research studies of the role of the ward sister, and the clinical area as a learning place, it is hoped to link learning with working, so that the nurse may become more alert to the vast number of learning opportunities that exist in the clinical area, and to how to create a climate where learning goes hand-in-hand with patient care, both being valued. These studies will be referred to and briefly described, so that the reader may gain an insight into the available research and can develop ideas, and gain hints and tips for learning, while working. Acknowledging that this book has been written for busy nurses, reference will be made, wherever possible, to published research in journal or monograph form; only if the research is not published will the original thesis be quoted. In order to introduce several aspects, reference to any one study is likely to be brief and will probably leave out interesting and relevant details. References will be given at the end of each chapter, in order to make it easier to follow them up, which the reader is strongly advised to do. If reading research reports or articles feels like trying to cope with a foreign language, there is a small booklet, *Reading Research*, which may help you (Ogier, 1989, Scutari Press). It does not provide all the answers, but is designed to provide help with reading research.

Examples will be taken from various nursing areas to try to relate theory and research findings to the work-place. It is advisable to try to find examples from your own nursing field to help you identify with the ideas discussed. Activities are also suggested at various points in the text, with the aim of helping you to relate what you read to your own work area.

Appendix I contains a minimal description of some educational theories, in order to provide the reader with a theoretical perspective upon which to relate the more practical aspects of this book. Appendixes II and III outline the British and American Codes of Practice.

The style of writing is informal, attempting to avoid educational and research jargon, and the book is viewed by the author as a 'warm-up' text for the busy nurse, who might otherwise not be interested in reading a more formal, detailed text. It is hoped that, having read this book, the reader will want to study in greater depth: a list of suggested publications for further reading will be found immediately before the Appendixes.

I am conscious that, in trying to write a text which is readable and short, the references to the many theories and research studies have not reflected adequately the expertise, skill, hard work and value of the writers of the works referred to. Likewise, the choice of works to which reference has been made reflects my preferences. There are other texts which another author might have preferred to include. I hope my efforts will help and motivate you to see the relevance of the reports to your work area and to willingly read more.

Margaret E Ogier
January 1989

Acknowledgements

This book would not have materialised if many nurses had not striven to seek the best for the profession and their fellow nurses on both sides of the Atlantic; thanks are due to many people, some unknown, who play their part in the complex nursing world.

Thanks to Hazel Allen and Christine Davies of the King's Fund Centre, who enabled researchers into the role of the ward sister to meet and compare and share their findings. Thanks to those researchers who shared so willingly, and whose studies have been inadequately referred to in this book – Margaret Alexander, Rosemary Bryant, Sally Farnish, Joan Fretwell, Judith Lathlean, Sheila Marson, Helen Orton, Sue Pembrey and Phil Runciman – and to the ward sisters in the UK and Eire who have been an inspiration for many of the ideas, without whose help this book would not be in existence. Thanks are also due to Rosemary White, who was the catalyst for this book being written.

I would also like to thank the editor, Patrick West, for his patience while the ideas germinated and spluttered into life, and for his constructive advice as the work progressed.

Thanks to Helen Litten for her willing and cheerful assistance with the mysteries of syntax and with the grammatical presentation of the manuscript, thus avoiding many split infinitives and the like!

Thanks go, too, to my long-suffering husband, who has been a tower of strength through my research and various professional activities, and who has provided sustained support throughout the struggles of this composition.

The letter by student nurse V Buxton, 'Being Honest on the Ward Report', is reproduced by kind permission of *Nursing Times*, where this letter first appeared on 18 November 1987.

Table 5.1 is also reproduced by kind permission of the *Nursing Times*. This table first appeared in the *Nursing Mirror* on 17 July 1985.

Thanks are also due to the American Nurses Association for permission to reproduce page 1 from *Code for Nurses with Interpretive Statements*, published in 1985 by the American Nurses Association, 2420 Pershing Road, Kansas City, Missouri, USA, and to the United Kingdom Central Council for Nursing, Midwifery and Health Visiting for permission to reproduce the *Code of Professional Conduct for the Nurse, Midwife and Health Visitor*, 2nd edition, November 1984.

I would like to thank: Lippincott/Harper and Row for permission to quote and use the work of C Breu and K Dracup, 'Implementing Nursing Research in Critical Care Settings', which appeared in the *Journal of Nursing Administration*, December 1976, pp. 14–17; John Wiley and Sons for permission to quote extracts from pp. 123–126 of D C Klein, *Community Dynamics in Mental Health*, published in 1968; and Prentice Hall for permission to use material from p. 15 of *Improving Leadership Performance* by P L Wright and D S Taylor.

Margaret E Ogier
January 1989

Introduction

This book has evolved from work carried out with experienced ward sisters and clinical nurses in the UK over the four years 1984–88. The ideas described have been reinforced by discussions in North America and by correspondence with a group of Icelandic nurses. The main focus of the work has been three-day workshops in different health authorities in England and Wales. The framework of the workshops comprises the research studies carried out since 1977 into the role of the ward sister. I am truly grateful to the researchers who have so willingly shared their findings and ideas, giving me the confidence to work with experienced nurses, helping them review their role in the ever-changing health-care field. I hope that you, the reader, will be able to gain an insight into the various research studies, and be stimulated to read more research as you begin to see the relevance of the findings to your work.

Many clinical nurses work extremely hard in the face of economic cutbacks, the changing demands of society and a need for increased professional awareness. They need help to release their enormous potential, which may have been restrained by prior *training*, resulting in unquestioning attitudes, adherence to policies, routinised care and a role as subservient 'doer' of the health-care team. Some of these closed, unthinking behaviours and attitudes have been reinforced by past traditions. The aim of this book is to help the busy nurse to renew her enthusiasm for learning as the means to better patient care and self-esteem, for, as Virginia Henderson wrote in her greeting to the international nursing research conference 'Clinical Excellence in Nursing: International Networking' held in Edinburgh in July 1987:

'When nurses' sensitivity to human need (their intuition) is joined with the ability to find and use expert opinion, with the ability to find reported research and apply it to their practice, and when they themselves use the scientific method of investigation, there is no limit to the influence they might have on health care worldwide.'

Nurses are frequently heard to say, 'I haven't the time to teach – I'm here to care for the patients!' This book is aimed at those nurses, to help them look at their role and function, and ensure that the care they work so hard to give is up to date and meeting the needs of the patients. Ideas will be considered on how they can help themselves and other nurses to be constantly alert to ways of improving care and developing greater job satisfaction. As nurses are required to be accountable for their decisions and actions, reference is made wherever possible to appropriate theories and research findings.

Chapter 1 will provide some background to the ideas and need for learning in the clinical area. Chapter 2 will look at research findings, particularly the research studies that relate to the role of the ward sister, head nurse or supervisor as they influence learning in the clinical area. In Chapter 3 an attempt is made to relate theory and research findings to practical suggestions for the busy nurse, with a view to enabling learning and teaching to progress in tandem with the everyday business of providing care. Chapter 4 follows with further practical tips. Chapter 5 will consider that learning may require change, and will discuss how change can be initiated, coped with and utilised for the benefit of nurse learning, as well as for improving patient well-being. The final chapter will consider a few topical issues and the future direction of nursing. Emphasis will be on the nurse as a self-directing, adult learner. Throughout the book suggestions for the reader's participation will be made, in the belief that, as adult learners, nurses will work to master what they see as relevant to their work. In the appendixes consideration will be made, briefly, to some theories of learning, in order to provide a framework upon which to consider learning in the clinical area.

It is suggested that readers should have a folder and some loose-leaf paper, on which to complete the exercises and record their ideas.

While this book is written for nurses, using nursing examples, it is anticipated that other health-care professionals will be able to identify with the philosophy expressed and gain by reading and inserting their own examples. Indeed, discussion with workers outside the health-care environment has revealed a need in several areas to facilitate learning in the work-place; I hope that some of the ideas will be of use, especially to the first-line manager and supervisor.

For ease of reading, I have used the word 'nurse' to mean the qualified nurse, and, in order to avoid infelicities of writing, I have adopted the convention that nurses are female, while recognising that many are male, and that patients are male, except where context dictates otherwise. 'Learner', 'nurse learner', 'student' and 'student nurse' refer to the person, male or female, who is following a nurse-education programme, bearing in mind that for professional expertise we are all learning all the time, and that a role as 'qualified nurse' cannot easily be separated from that of 'learner'.

1
Learning in the Clinical Area

The aim of this chapter is to consider why there should be learning in the clinical area. Four broad themes run through it, related to the need to learn. These are:

- society's expectations;
- the requirements of the trained nurse;
- the needs of the student nurse following a basic education programme;
- the personal satisfaction and growth experienced through learning.

INTRODUCTION

'Whatever competence means today we can be sure its meaning will have changed by tomorrow. The foundation for future professional competence seems to be the capacity to learn how to learn. (Schein, 1972, quoted in Argyris and Schön, 1976)

Surely, there can be little argument that a great change is taking place in nursing and related professions. In the UK, there is a major review of basic and post-basic nurse education, the National Health Service has been 'reorganised' for the third time in recent years, and medical advances continue, with the development of more intricate technology. A similar story is heard in Australia, where some states have removed nurse training from hospitals to higher education establishments, with resulting implications not only for nurse education, but also for manpower in hospitals and the community. Changes are taking place in North American nursing, as the role of the nurse alters to meet changing demands. Concurrent with all these changes, there is a growing awareness that only a limited supply of money is available to meet ever-expanding health needs. Nurses are at the meeting place of limited resources and patients' needs. They are where available resources are deployed, and will be expected by managers and administrators to be economical and

1

cost-conscious, while patients and clients and their relatives will expect the best possible care to meet their needs.

Since nurses have limited resources of time, manpower and money at their disposal, how do they assess the situation and plan to meet needs which frequently appear greater than resources? The need for nurses to continue learning and developing the skills necessary to meet new challenges, not just in health care but in associated areas such as management, financial control and political power, is clear, and is common to most countries of the world. One hopes that the cry, 'But we have always done it that way!', when some long-cherished ritual is questioned, will soon be gone. Rather, nurses will be able to give a knowledgeable account of their decision-making and be accountable for their nursing prescriptions and actions.

SOCIETY'S EXPECTATIONS

Society's needs and expectations are ever changing, not only due to changing disease patterns and altered affluence, but also because the public is increasingly better informed by the mass media, and made more aware of the latest treatments and medical ideas. This increased public awareness may result in unrealistic demands on the health services for treatments and cures that are not readily available, either owing to their cost or because they are still at the developmental stage. Increased public awareness may also bring undue fear and anxiety, for information may be misunderstood or poorly understood, as, for example, when AIDS was brought to the attention of the public with a view to preventing its spread and, through fear and lack of understanding, several potential sufferers were treated like outcasts and children excluded from school.

Well, what has that got to do with you as a nurse? I am sure some of you will have experienced the double standards set for you by neighbours and friends. From the day on which you started nurse training, some of them regarded you as the fount of all wisdom on health matters, expecting you to diagnose little Johnny's spots and to know what to do about Granny's lumps and bumps, while others were quite amazed that you had to set aside time to study and pass examinations: 'After all, we thought you were going to be a nurse and care for people! What's that bookwork got to do with washing and feeding people?'

So how do you cope with these contradictory expectations? For a start, I do not suggest that you become the fount of all wisdom. Recently, I was given one of those plastic place-mats with an animal picture and a 'wise saying'; the picture was of a small, forlorn-looking kitten, which had got stuck in the top of a milk jug. The 'saying' was 'Half of being smart is knowing what you're dumb at'. For the sake of young Johnny, Granny and the public at large, we as nurses need to know our limitations, and be aware of topics of current interest and to whom to refer for accurate advice and information. We also need to be aware of professional and political issues that affect those for whom we care in both our private and professional lives. However, this book will not dwell on aspects of political awareness, which is now an essential part of a nurse's repertoire, since excellent texts have already been written in this area (Salvage, 1985; White, 1985, 1986, 1988; Clay, 1987). Every trained nurse needs to be aware of issues beyond the bedside, which directly affect the care she gives, for as White (1985) said:

'Decision making has, therefore, assumed greater meaning and now takes place at a distance from the practitioner: it involves the government bureaucracy and political and fiscal considerations. Nursing is now shaped by politics but we have been slow to accept these factors and to develop a more sophisticated and worldly understanding of them.'

Professional bodies require trained nurses to be competent and up to date. The United Kingdom Central Council for Nursing, Midwifery and Health Visiting (UKCC, 1984) Code of Professional Conduct (see Appendix II) states:

'Each registered nurse, midwife and health visitor is accountable for his or her practice, and, in the exercise of professional accountability shall:

'3. Take every reasonable opportunity to maintain and improve professional knowledge and competence.'

The American Nurses Association (1985) Code for Nurses with Interpretive Statements (see Appendix III) states:

'5.1 The profession of nursing is obligated to provide adequate and competent nursing care. Therefore it is the personal responsibility of each nurse to maintain competency in practice . . .

' . . .The nurse must be aware of the need for continued professional learning and must assume personal responsibility for currency of knowledge and skills.'

REQUIREMENTS OF THE TRAINED NURSE

Who learns what from whom and how?

Exercise

Before I share some ideas with you, take a sheet of paper and write down what *you* think you can learn in and from the work-place, be it ward, theatre, community or residential home.

Some of the things on your list may apply to other trained nurses. The UKCC Code of Conduct requires us to assist our peers, that is our equals, and our subordinates to develop competence in accordance with their needs. Underline those items on your list that may apply to other trained nurses with whom you work. Now stop, think and list any other learning opportunities that there may be for your peers and subordinates in the work-place.

First, what can be learnt or developed in the clinical area? Broadly speaking, *knowledge, skills* and *attitudes* related to the specific area can be assimilated.

Let us take an example which may be relevant to most countries.

Mr. Jamie Peterson is 58 and is a storekeeper who lives alone, having been divorced five years ago. He has developed a varicose ulcer on his right leg, which causes him much pain and which, despite several visits to his doctor and different treatments, has gradually worsened. Eventually, Mr Peterson has agreed to take a week off work to rest his leg, and the doctor has arranged for the nurse to make home visits and dress the ulcer.

Some of the abilities and behaviours required by the community nurse visiting Mr Peterson include:

Knowledge of:

- the latest occlusive dressing for varicose ulcers;
- the pathology and healing process of such ulcers;
- society's pressures on Mr Peterson to behave or conform in certain ways, which may not be best for his health; for example he may drink to excess to be 'one of the boys'.

The *skills* to:

- apply the appropriate dressing correctly;
- gain Mr Peterson's co-operation.

The *attitude* of:

- caring concern for the pain and disability caused by the ulcer and how these may affect his life-style and well-being.

The nurse will also need the skills of a *teacher* to educate Mr Peterson, so that he will rest with his leg raised.

The nurse may have to call upon her knowledge of different forms of *communication* and upon all her *interpersonal skills*, in order to make sure that Mr Peterson hears and understands the need for co-operation in his treatment.

The nurse may need to *negotiate* with the doctor for a change of treatment or relevant prescription; negotiation may entail her in demonstrating her knowledge of:

- the care of the individual patient with the varicose ulcer;
- the effects of the proposed treatment;
- the *cost* and *benefits*, in terms of materials, nurse's time, patient's time off work, etc.

The nurse has to *manage* her workload, in order to ensure that the necessary care is given. This entails *identifying priorities*, *decision-making skills*, and *teaching and supervision* of other staff, patient and relatives, all with different needs and expectations.

I hope that this small example has highlighted the enormous range of topics and skills which can be studied or developed in the clinical area. I am sure that you will have included examples of similar activities and learning opportunities in your lists.

Second, who learns?

Exercise

Considering the above example, make a list of the people who may learn from Mr Peterson's problem. Then read on.

The *nurse* may learn:

- from the patient, about his life-style and needs related to treatment of the ulcer;

- from the various suppliers of occlusive dressings;
- from tutors or from pharmaceutical representatives on a study day or visit to a specialist area;
- from other nurses who have found a particular treatment beneficial;
- from journals;
- from the doctor.

In addition, the nurse may learn from managers or administrators about budgeting and how to make her activities cost effective. She may learn bargaining and negotiating skills directly from seniors or union representatives, or indirectly through role-modelling.

One hopes that the *patient* will learn from the nurse about self-care and the prevention of illness or, at least, how not to aggravate his ulcer.

The *doctor* may learn from the nurse's expertise in a particular area, and of how she can contribute to the well-being of patients and clients.

Other nurses may copy the nurse who acts as a role model, with a sound knowledge base, relevant clinical skills, skills of acting as the patient's advocate, budgeting and bargaining acumen, and a caring attitude that values the individual's rights.

It can be seen at a glance that the work-place is also one vast area in which to learn and develop a whole range of knowledge, skills and attitudes – clinical, managerial and professional.

Stapleton (1982) explored the views of trained nurses in one health authority in the south of England regarding the need for continuing education. She gave questionnaires to 284 charge nurses and nursing officers to ascertain their views on continuing professional development, with the result that:

- 94% of nurses felt some need to update;
- 27% of those nurses felt a *great* need to update.

Her study showed that nurses were aware of the need for continuing education, but that difficulties existed in finding ways of meeting the need. The nurses placed emphasis for continuing education on activities outside the clinical area. Both Runciman (1982) and Stapleton (1982) concluded that there was a need for education within the clinical setting.

A recent study by Rogers and Lawrence (1987) looked at continuing professional education for nurses, midwives and health visitors in England and Wales. The aims of the study were to examine the current provision for continuing professional education for qualified nurses, to explore nurses' perceptions of continuing education related to their work, and to establish how nurses' needs were identified. The study consisted of two phases. Phase One was a survey of opportunities for continuing professional education, and Phase Two a case study in depth of two health districts. Rogers and Lawrence found that while there was verbal commitment to continuing professional education in the majority of health authorities, there was little practical provision such as budgeted money. Manpower planning did not include study leave, and there were no written educational philosophies for continuing education available to individual nurses. Indeed, one unexpected outcome of the survey was that many chief nursing officers said that their awareness of the need to provide continuing education had been raised following the request to provide information for the study.

Rogers and Lawrence also found that the needs of continuing professional education fall into one of four main areas:

- The individual nurse's professional development needs
- The individual nurse's personal development needs
- The development needs of the particular clinical area in which the nurse is working
- The longer-term needs of the health authority, as identified in strategic and operational plans

One of Rogers and Lawrence's recommendations is that it is important to develop the individual's commitment to self-development, and that the individual should understand that she has a joint responsibility with the employing authority to ensure that continuing education occurs.

Another important aspect of qualified nurses' learning considered by Rogers and Lawrence is an issue that is likely to increase in importance over the next few years – the shortage of 18-year-olds and a shortfall in recruitment to nurse training. The authors highlight the importance of attracting qualified nurses back into nursing and the need to provide suitable education for them. How important it is that the nurse returning after a break of years from the clinical area should return to an area where there is a clear mandate for learning, and to an environment in which it will be safe to voice anxieties and gain confidence! Returning nurses will need help to refresh and build on their existing knowledge, develop new skills and review attitudes.

It may be in the area of professional attitudes that the biggest change has taken place or is taking place, as nurses become primary care givers, make nursing assessments, prescribe nursing care and are accountable for their decisions and actions. Nursing no longer has a subservient role, but rather is a partner in care, a partner to the doctor, paramedic and administrator. Many, many nurses in and returning to practice are going to need all the support they can get from the clinical environment, in order to learn and grow, and thus take on the mantle of partner, not servant.

Rogers and Lawrence (1987), interviewing trained nurses, found that, when newly qualified, only just over half of them (58%) turned to senior trained colleagues for help and support. However, when in post, 82% of qualified nurses looked to senior colleagues for help and support. When qualified nurses were asked about the perceived relevance of continuing education:

- 55% said it was useful to exchange ideas and that it made them think;
- 17% said it was directly relevant to their clinical work;
- 27% did not find it had any use or relevance to clinical work.

(Percentages have been rounded to whole numbers and, therefore, total 99%).

When interviewed about other ways of helping themselves to keep up to date:

- 28% said they read a nursing journal;
- 39% took part in informal discussion groups;
- 6% attended professional organisation study days;
- 11% followed up their own interests;
- 15% had no additional involvement with continuing professional education.

Some of the sisters found that having nurses in training allocated to their areas stimulated them to keep up to date. Similar views are often expressed by sisters attending the writer's three-day Sister Development Workshops. The sisters comment that having learner nurses who question makes one stop and think. So, what are the needs of the nurses in training?

THE NEEDS OF THE NURSE IN TRAINING

Nurses in training also work in the clinical area: whether they are following a degree programme, a baccalaureate scheme or an apprenticeship type of training, there comes a point when experience has to be gained in the clinical area – how important it is to ensure that this is a learning experience as well!

Exercise

List all the learning opportunities for a nurse in training which are available in your work areas. Now look through your list and group together similar items – e.g. wound care, removal of sutures and removal of clips are all procedures requiring an aseptic technique. This will help to identify the common types of opportunity available in your area, and facilitate comparison with other nurses' perceptions.

If you have student nurses gaining experience with you, ask each of them to make a list of the learning they hope to achieve during the experience.

Now compare your list with theirs. Look at the similarities in the lists and discuss with the students how the opportunities can be utilised. Explore with the students where there are differences. Are the differences merely semantic – different words being used to describe the same thing – or are there real differences? Are the students unaware of what is available to them, or do they have unrealistic expectations? Are there aspects you had not considered as relevant or as learning opportunities? As we become more experienced it is easy to take for granted certain aspects that may be novel, difficult or even alarming for the student new to the area.

Keep the lists by you, as you will need them for the next exercise.

By being willing to ask students their views, and by exploring with them their needs and expectations, you have demonstrated that you regard them as intelligent adults, responsible for their own learning. You will also have shown that you are approachable, thereby developing a climate of good rapport and two-way communication.

Up to now, nurse training in the UK might be regarded as being of the apprenticeship type, in which the nurse spends most of her training time working in clinical areas. A review of the literature related to nurse training is provided by Jacka and

Lewin (1987). Proposals are being put forward (UKCC, 1987) for the nurse in training to have student status and be supernumerary to the staff in the clinical area. However, whatever type of education programme prevails, the clinical area needs to be conducive to learning. Let us now consider, 'What learning?'

When beginning my research into the role of the ward sister and how she can make or mar learning in the wards, I spent some time talking to my colleagues about my ideas. One informal debate over coffee was about whether or not it mattered what the nurse wanted to learn, because the sister 'knew best', she was the one with experience and knew what had to be learnt for patient safety. One sister in charge of a thoracic ward required all student nurses working in her ward to demonstrate by the end of two weeks' experience the safe care of a patient undergoing underwater seal drainage. The sister outlined the crucial aspects of ensuring that the bottle was not knocked over or emptied, that it was not raised above the level of the bed, and so on, and many other points which could put the safety of the patient at risk if the nurse was unaware of them; therefore, the need was to ensure that the nurse learnt swiftly and accurately. None of those present at the discussion wished to disagree about the importance of the issues which she raised, but some were concerned that there were many other valuable learning opportunities in that busy ward, and that the sister should not lose sight of these in her anxiety to ensure safe nursing care for patients with underwater seal drainage. As a result of that discussion, I became concerned that there might be a mismatch between the nurse's expectation of what she could learn in a particular allocation and the expectations of the sister or nurse in charge, responsible for what the nurse should be learning. That is why I have just asked you to list the learning opportunities in your work area, and then to ask the nurses in training to list the opportunities that they were expecting. Do the lists match? If they do, all well and good! If they do not, at least you are aware of a mismatch of perceptions and can begin to resolve any major differences.

As a result of my concern, I arranged to ask groups of nurses in training to list what they wanted to learn in their next placement. I also asked groups of sisters and staff nurses, all in general hospitals, what learning opportunities were available in their clinical areas. The results were as follows:

- 193 nurses in training mentioned 740 learning opportunities that they were expecting from their next placements; each nurse knew to where she was allocated.

- 55 staff nurses identified 305 learning opportunities in their areas.
- 23 sisters also identified 97 learning opportunities.

The sisters and staff nurses identified more opportunities than did the nurses in training; the mean number of items for sisters was 4.2, for staff nurses, 5.5, and for nurses in training, 3.8.

You might think it was to be expected that the experienced nurses would be aware of what was to be learnt. By a process of content analysis, common themes in the responses were identified, and it was possible to include all the opportunities under one of five headings:

1. *Theory*, 'to know about': 'I want to learn more about care of patients with heart failure.'
2. *Practical*, the 'to do' category: 'I want to learn how to do a wound dressing.'
3. *Ward climate*: 'I want to work in a ward where I am not made to feel stupid if I don't know something', 'I want to be made to feel *part* of the ward team'.
4. *Accessories*: 'I want to work where there are books to look things up in, or charts to explain things.'
5. *Miscellaneous*: 'I'd like to see some of our local housing – then I might understand why Mrs Smith never has a bath.'

The predominant categories were theory and practical. If we look at these two categories:

- students mentioned theory 248 times and practical 241 times;
- staff nurses mentioned theory 97 times and practical 73 times;
- sisters mentioned theory 14 times and practical 35 times.

Thus, it can be seen at a glance that theory and practical learning opportunities are of equal importance to nurses in training. However, staff nurses identify more opportunities 'to learn about' (theory), than 'to do' (practical), while the sisters' emphasis is on practical opportunities. Is this a potential area for mismatch of expectations, the nurse in training seeking as much theoretical information as practical opportunities from the work-place, with sisters only identifying one theoretical opportunity to every 2.5 practical opportunities? As my research progressed, this was to prove to be one of the aspects which could result in a sister making or marring a learning experience in the clinical area (see Ogier, 1983, for a more detailed account). Are you placing the same emphasis on learning various aspects as are the students in training?

Before we leave the topic of checking presumptions of what someone else needs to know, let me share another point with you about the information-gathering stage of the research just described. I believe that it is essential to provide feedback to anyone who has helped to complete questionnaires or answer questions during a research project. Six groups of nurses, who were representative of those at the beginning, middle and the end of training, provided information on what kind of learning opportunities they had expected to encounter in their next clinical placement. For each group the emphasis remained on theory and practical, as the overall figures show. The nurses who were midway in their training generated fewer items than those at the beginning or end; this possibly reflects the dip which occurs in the middle of any training for, as they explained to me, 'Well, we are over the enthusiasm of the start, and finals are still a way off'. The nurses at the end of training were due to sit their final examinations in six weeks' time. I had presumed that the overall balance of an equal amount of theory to practical would be the result of beginners wanting practical experience and the finalists a lot of theory. To my amazement, the finalists were looking for more practical learning opportunities than were any other group of nurses in training. I was keen to return to them with the findings and to hear their explanations, which were that they were so near to finals that what they did not know by then was too late to worry about. 'But why so much practical', I asked, 'You have been nursing for three years – surely you are competent in many aspects of care?' They replied that, as senior student nurses, they often acted up for the staff nurse, and they hoped that they would be qualified nurses in a few weeks: 'There is nothing like having to show a junior nurse how to do something to make you realise the importance of doing it properly.' Therefore, the senior student nurses were anxious to practise and perfect their practical skills.

Jacka and Lewin (1987) found that the first-year student nurses who were involved in their study mainly worked with third-year student nurses or enrolled nurses. When asked to rate how often practical demonstrations occurred, on a scale of 'often', 'sometimes', 'rarely' or 'never', most students said 'sometimes'. The practical demonstrations varied from the administration of medicines to applying aseptic dressings, the instillation of eye drops and last offices. Using the same rating scale, students were asked how often their theoretical knowledge was questioned; again, the main response was 'sometimes', but responses varied widely. Patients in the wards were a rich source of clinical material, upon which the students' theoretical knowledge was questioned, students being asked to explain the reason for a particular nursing action, or the different kinds of operation available for a specific condition. How patients adapted to disease or to a prosthesis was also a rich source of questioning. Jacka and Lewin propose that learning is likely to increase with the frequency of demonstration or questioning by trained nurses. The same students indicated few obvious impediments to learning; although they were aware of shortcomings in their education programme, they were not dissatisfied with their training.

Jacka and Lewin also asked student nurses and sisters to rate the ward as a learning experience for student nurses, on a scale from 1 (the experience taught them very little) to 10 (the experience taught them a great deal). The mean for the students' rating of the wards was 7.4, with a maximum of 10 and a minimum of 1.8. The mean for the sisters' rating was 8.2, and the sisters saw the wards as providing more learning than was perceived by the student nurses.

Student nurses almost certainly have learning objectives. You may have been involved in setting the objectives, but this is not always so. Look at the objectives and note how many relate to theory and how many to practical experience.

Exercise

In a previous exercise, you and the student nurses made lists of the learning opportunities available in your area; now compare those lists with the learning objectives of the student nurses. Are they similar? Do they cover the same topics?

If not, should one or the other be altered to bring perceived needs, as identified by the learning opportunities, into line with required needs as listed in the learning objectives? Now approach the originator of the objectives, with a view to negotiating mutually acceptable objectives that reflect the available opportunities.

Finally, why should there be all this learning? My personal philosophy in connection with nurse education is that a nurse will work at and put effort into mastering knowledge and skills that can be seen to be relevant to patient care and well-being. This is based on personal experience, but is reinforced by the writings of Rogers (1983) and Knowles (1984). Jacka and Lewin (1987) write that there has been concern for many years about the adequacy of the clinical education received by student nurses. Few guidelines have been available to assist those concerned with improving the educational quality of the clinical allocation, and, while this book does not claim to provide those missing guidelines, it is hoped that the following chapters may provide some hints and tips for increasing the educational value of the work-place.

Having now briefly considered society's expectations, professional requirements and training needs, let us turn to the need for personal growth and development.

PERSONAL GROWTH AND SATISFACTION THROUGH LEARNING

I hope that you will be convinced from the title of the book and the preceding paragraphs that the learning being considered is very different from the schooling which many of us received – seated behind a desk, often learning by rote and not deviating from the topic or lesson content. Learning should be lively and stimulating, not necessarily easy but meaningful, so that the time, energy and effort put into it will make the whole seem worth while, both for teacher and learner. From the learning can come personal growth and improved care for the patients and clients. To conclude this chapter, what better than to quote from an editorial written by Baroness Cox (1984):

> 'Learning does require courage – it may shatter complacency, discover disturbing facts, and require us to reappraise current ideas and policies. But we can be helped to "have the courage to learn" by sharing our knowledge and experience, reassured that we all share the same goal – the enhancement of standards of nursing practice and of nursing's contribution to the provision of health care.'

Rogers and Lawrence (1987) identified the most important aspect of work for the trained nurse as being patient care: 53% of the nurses interviewed responded that patient care was their priority, but the proportion did vary with the grade of the nurse. Ward sisters placed equal emphasis on patient care and on management. Bevis (1975), quoted by Rogers and Lawrence, demonstrated that the nurses with the highest loyalty to patient care were those most likely to participate in continuing education. It is important to bear this in mind when nurses say that they took up nursing to be with the patient, and appear reluctant to take part in any form of educational activity. If they are concerned for the patient, they should be seeking every opportunity to increase their expertise, and to ensure that the care which they prescribe and give is soundly based and up to date. The confidence of giving effective care based on a framework of up-to-date knowledge, skilled, competent perform-ance and professional attitudes enhances the individual nurse's well-being.

Learning not only enhances professional competence and the satisfaction of care well given, but also increases personal growth and self-esteem, which are essential for the nurse as a whole person. At a time when there is a shortage of nurses, coupled with difficulty in retaining qualified staff, the value of a stimulating, educationally orientated work-place cannot be overlooked for the well-being of the individual nurse, the organisation and the patient.

References

American Nurses Association (1985) *Code for Nurses with Interpretive Statements.* Kansas City, Missouri: American Nurses Association.

Argyris C and Schön D A (1976) *Theory in Practice: Increasing Professional Effectiveness.* San Francisco: Jossey-Bass.

Clay T (1987) *Nurses, Power and Politics.* London: Heinemann.

Cox C (1984) Editorial. Special issues, developments in nursing education. *International Journal of Nursing Studies*, 21(13): 151–152.

Jacka K and Lewin D (1987) *The Clinical Learning of Student Nurses.* NERU Report No. 6. London: Nursing Education Research Unit, King's College, University of London.

Knowles M (1984) *The Adult Learner: A Neglected Species*, 3rd edn. Houston: Gulf Publishing Co.

Ogier M E (1983) The ward sister as a teacher resource person. In: *Research into Nurse Education*, ed. Davis B D. London: Croom Helm.

Rogers C R (1983) *Freedom to Learn for the Eighties.* Columbus, Ohio: Charles E Merril.

Rogers J and Lawrence J (1987) *Continuing Professional Education for Qualified Nurses, Midwives and Health Visitors. A Report of a Survey and Case Study.* Peterborough: Ashdale Press.

Runciman P J (1982) Ward sisters: their problems at work – 1 and 2. *Nursing Times*, Occasional Papers, **78** (36 & 37): 141–144, 145–147.

Salvage J (1985) *The Politics of Nursing.* London: Heinemann.

Stapleton M F (1982) Update, top-ranking. *Nursing Mirror*, March 24: 38–40.

United Kingdom Central Council for Nursing, Midwifery and Health Visiting (1984) *Code of Conduct for the Nurse, Midwife and Health Visitor.* London: UKCC.

United Kingdom Central Council for Nursing, Midwifery and Health Visiting (1987) *Project 2000: The Final Proposals. Project Paper 9.* London: UKCC.

White R (1985) *Political Issues in Nursing: Past, Present and Future, Vol. 1.* Chichester: John Wiley and Sons.

White R (1986) *Political Issues in Nursing: Past, Present and Future, Vol. 2.* Chichester: John Wiley and Sons.

White R (1988) *Political Issues in Nursing: Past, Present and Future, Vol. 3.* Chichester: John Wiley and Sons.

2
Creating a Learning Environment in the Clinical Area

As indicated at the end of the last chapter, learning in the work area may be very different from that experienced in school, or even in nurse training. During the last decade, it was recognised in industry and in general education that adults learn best when the topic is related to their needs, and that when experience can be linked with present learning, development of the individual is then likely to take place. The National Health Service Training Authority reports, in *Better Management, Better Health* (1986):

'It has been shown that managers tend to learn more effectively if there are clear cycles connecting theory with practice. This means firm links between what a manager already knows through experience, the opportunity to learn new insights, concepts or skills, and then the reinforcement/refinement of that learning through subsequent experience.'

Whether holding a formal management position, such as that of ward sister, or not, all nurses are managers of patient care, and this management element is likely to increase for every nurse as the profession moves nearer to primary nursing. Let us now look at a few theories of learning, as these support a person's work as a nurse. Without motivation and commitment however, all efforts to learn and develop will come to naught. Jacka and Lewin (1987) asked ward sisters which of all the factors they would rate as most important in helping them in their teaching role. Their responses showed that the two most important factors were students who were keen to learn and staff who were keen to teach. Hall et al wrote in 1981:

'Unless the people who have contact with the patient have sufficient commitment, motivation, satisfaction and adjustment to the organisation, the effects of professional preparation and knowledge may be mitigated or obliterated entirely.'

Redfern (1980) reports that intrinsic satisfaction had no effect on whether or not hospital sisters stayed in post; rather, it was the extrinsic satisfaction, such as opportunities for advancement, hospital policies and practices, supervision and recognition which attracted them. So, while sisters were committed to nursing, they left because they were disenchanted with their working environment.

Some of the nursing research findings about the work situation that is also a learning environment will be considered later in this chapter. However, it is necessary first of all to consider what is meant by learning. Rather than bewilder the reader with a resumé of all the possible theories, Knowles (1984) lists 86 educational theorists who, between 1885 and 1980, put forward various suppositions related to learning. A definition of learning is given below, and some of the theories which may seem particularly pertinent to nursing and learning in the clinical area can be found in Appendix I. Any reader wishing to delve into the theoretical aspects of learning is referred to Quinn (1988), Child (1986), Jarvis (1983) or Van Hoozer et al (1987).

What is learning? Knowles (1984) reviews 18 definitions of learning, but, as these are debated at length in the textbooks just referred to, it is unnecessary to consider them here or to choose between them. The definition that will be used from now on in this book is: *Learning is a change in knowledge, skills and/or attitudes as the result of experience* (James, 1970). Therefore, how can one best ensure that the nursing experience is also a learning experience, and that what is learnt is desirable and not the copying of bad habits or incorrect procedures?

Experience consists of several parts or facets:

- the situation itself, e.g. the wound dressing or helping an anxious patient to explore the nature of his anxiety;
- the organisation or context in which the experience is occurring, e.g. the hospital, the ward or the patient's home;
- the participants in the experience, e.g. the patient or client, the relatives, the ward sister and/or the staff nurse.

As described in Chapter 1 when considering Mr Peterson, all participants will be learning something, whether or not they are conscious of it, or whether or not it is what they should be learning.

From this it can be seen that for desired learning to take place, several aspects have to be considered and, as far as possible, planned and/or controlled. To begin with, consider where the experience is taking place and the organisational climate.

Fretwell (1980a), reporting on her research into the ward learning environment, writes that where there was a rigid routine, the spirit of enquiry was stifled, and this affected individualised patient care. Fretwell describes how nurses regard much of nursing as basic work, repetitive and not related to their education. She quotes a first year student nurse:

'I suppose learning is reinforced every time we do something, but on some wards you fall into the routine and don't think about it.'

How does learning theory fit the organisation's management philosophy? Revans wrote in 1961:

'Where a sister's view of the hospital organisation is that it is forthcoming toward her problems, and where her views upon seniority, status and authority are flexible, then her outlook upon the student nurse is likely to be sympathetic; where, on the contrary, her opinion is that the hospital organisation is aloof or even hostile, or where she herself has authoritarian views upon codes of hospital precedence, her attitude towards nurse training is likely to be indifferent or even disparaging.'

It is to be hoped that training for management in the NHS will now reflect the value of experience, creating a learning environment in the clinical area that is person-centred and experiential, so that too much dissonance or tension will not occur. The National Health Service Training Authority's Report (1986) says:

'Developing managers often means starting from where they are "at". It means using the managers' real world issues and problems as the basis on which to build ... NHS managers should search out good learning designs which relate to the real issues being explored.'

In the real world of patient care, this is what nurse educationalists working with trained nurses have been doing for several years (Pembrey, 1980; Marson, 1982; Farnish, 1983; Lathlean et al, 1986; Ogier, 1986; Lathlean, 1988). Perhaps managers in the health service will become conversant with creating a learning environment in the work-place, so that efforts to create a learning environment in the clinical area will be compatible with organisational philosophy, and so that the rigid unyielding system that previously encompassed health care will be a thing of the past. For as Knowles (1984) writes:

'... there is a need for both the direct facilitation of the development of individuals and the indirect facilitation of their development through improving the educative quality of their environments.'

Having considered briefly the learning experience as part of a larger organisational structure, it is necessary to consider the individuals involved in this experience. When demonstrating how to cleanse a wound to a first year student nurse, who is doing the learning and what is being learnt? One hopes that it is the student, but how about the person demonstrating the technique? Is it just another dressing technique to be demonstrated yet again, or can there be learning and development of skills in teaching, of interpersonal skills, and so on? Surely this nurse is different from the one taught yesterday? Even the shortage of nurses has not yet resulted in clones! And what was the patient learning?

One theoretical perspective of learning which relates well to the humanistic art of nursing is that of Rogers (1983). He believes that individuals have a natural potential to learn and will learn when the subject matter is seen to be relevant. Fretwell (1980a) reported that nurses caring for a patient having peritoneal dialysis could immediately identify that learning had taken place; new techniques have been mastered because these are essential to the care of that patient. Readers will know of nurses who have not fully understood and internalised the philosophy of individualised patient care – the nursing process – because they cannot see that it is different in any way from what they always do and regard it as just a paper exercise. Rogers also considers that much significant learning is acquired through doing. Certainly, this concept is of relevance to nursing, much of which is of a practical nature, and is of importance to the consideration of learning in the work-place. He also proposes that self-initiated learning involving the whole person, feelings as well as intellect, is the most pervasive and lasting.

Exercise

Stop and think of your most vivid learning experience during your training. Why is it the most memorable? Jot down a few notes about it, how you felt, what happened and what you learnt. Ask a student or colleague to do likewise. Then look for common themes and feelings that you both may have had. This may help you to identify some issue that can affect learning in the clinical area.

Chapter 1 considered what was to be learnt in the work-place: in general, knowledge, skills and attitudes related to clinical expertise, management, education and professional issues.

Exercise

Prepare a grid similar to the one shown below and complete the grid with examples of what you can learn in your work-place.

	Clinical	*Managerial*	*Professional*
Knowledge			
Skills			
Attitudes			

You may like to ask one or two of your colleagues or peers to complete a similar grid; you can then compare how perspectives of the same work-place may vary in relation to needs and experience.

Now, some of the research findings on the role of the ward sister will be discussed.

In order that learning may take place, the clinical area has to be managed by a leader who is in touch with the needs and abilities of her subordinates, and who is able to create an atmosphere which is conducive to learning. Some of the organisational constraints have already been discussed; now the role of the ward sister, the key to successful management of the clinical area, will be considered, by looking at different aspects in turn.

The ward sister can be viewed as:

- manager (Pembrey, 1980);
- leader (Ogier, 1982);
- teacher (Fretwell, 1982, 1985; Marson, 1982; Bryant, 1985);
- creator of a learning environment (Orton, 1981).

Reference will also be made to other studies and reports related to nurses, management and learning. For ease of comprehension, each issue will be dealt with separately, but cross-referencing is inevitable and, in real life, the aspects are interwoven and interconnected. Although the emphasis is on the ward sister as head of the nursing team, the material discussed is of relevance to any trained nurse.

In a report on the clinical learning of student nurses, Jacka and Lewin (1987) say that the problems of clinical learning are similar, regardless of type of hospital, training scheme or geographical location (all in the UK). They found that student nurses were effective estimators of their experience in the ward. Students were asked to rate their current ward placement as a learning environment. The behaviour and attitude of trained staff appeared to be the discriminating element. In highly rated wards the trained staff gave more practical demonstrations, worked more with students, supervised them more and were more approachable. These sisters were typically older, more experienced, better qualified and more openly committed to teaching.

Consideration of various aspects of the role of the trained nurse in creating a learning environment in the clinical area has been carried out in the UK by Orton (1981), Fretwell (1982, 1985), Marson (1982), Ogier (1982, 1986), Reid (1985). In North America, Layton (1969) endeavoured to identify which behaviours of instructors helped or hindered nurse students. She found that the behaviour that most affected students, by helping or hindering, was the instructor's reaction to the student as a person. More recently, Buccheri (1986) wrote that a supportive supervisor is a nurse who assists other nurses to meet their need for influence, communication and recognition. Supportive supervisors also share information and encourage those whom they supervise to share in the organisation.

Marson (1982) points out that:

' . . . on the job teaching of nurses is a complex global act in which the role model presented has a powerful influence . . .'.

Some of the findings related to the 'compex global act' will now be considered.

THE SISTER AS MANAGER

The purpose of Pembrey's (1980) study was to develop measures of ward sister performance in relation to individualised nursing, with a view to identifying behaviours that could be used to assess and train sisters. She used the four activities of the management cycle to assess whether sisters were managers. The four activities of the management cycle are assessing the situation, planning, carrying out the plan and checking that the implemented plan meets the requirements identified by the assessment. Nurses are now famliar with these four activities in terms of the nursing process:

- Assess.
- Plan.
- Implement.
- Evaluate.

For the purpose of the research study, Pembrey looked at four nursing activities, which can be taken to represent the four activities of the management of nursing and patient care, regardless of whether primary nursing care, patient allocation or team nursing is practised. These four activities are:

- the nursing round of patients;
- verbal work prescription;
- verbal allocation of nurses;
- accountability reports.

Fifty ward sisters were involved in the study, and were asked to rank 12 daily work priorities in order of importance. The activities ranked most important were:

- doing a ward round of the patients;
- giving the nurses a report on the patients;
- checking that the student nurses were managing their work.

However, asking nurses to report on their work ranked only sixth. It can be seen that the 50 sisters identified the first two activities of the management cycle as being important, and that the final part, accountability, did not feature highly.

These priorities were what the sisters *said* they rated as being the most important, but Pembrey also observed the sisters in order to establish whether or not they were doing what they said. Of the 50 sisters:

- only 17 did a complete nursing round of the patients;
- 23 did an incomplete round;
- 10 did no round.

Yet this activity was given the greatest verbal priority. Furthermore:

- 9 sisters gave verbal work prescription;
- 10 sisters verbally allocated nurses;
- 5 sisters received accountability reports.

Pembrey concludes that only 5 out of 50 sisters were managing patient care!

Why does it matter whether sisters manage patient care? What has that got to do with working and learning? In order to answer these questions, let us look at two of the sisters whom Pembrey observed, one who completed the cycle of management activities and another who did not, and whose clinical areas were as similar as possible in the number of staff, beds and so on.

Pembrey compares the percentage of the day spent by each sister in certain activities (Table 2.1). (Only the activities relevant to the discussion are depicted in the table; therefore, they do not total 100%. For a complete analysis see Pembrey, 1980.)

Table 2.1 Percentage of sister's day spent in defined activities

	Managing sister	Non-managing sister
Managing nursing	20%	1%
Working with patients alone	5%	19%
Working with patients and nurses	12%	3%

The managing sister spent 20% of her day in managing the nursing team, as compared with the 1% spent by the non-managing sister. This might be expected by the definition used for the selection of the sisters, but what does it mean in real work and learning terms? If the nursing team is not managed, it implies that there may be no assessment of patient needs, staff abilities and needs, and no allocation of nurses to patients or even to tasks. Pembrey found, in the wards where little or no management was practised, that at the end of the shift some patients had received no nursing, yet some nurses had been underoccupied.

Sisters and staff nurses attending workshops to develop their teaching and management skills commonly say, 'We came into nursing to nurse patients, not to be shut away in an office doing paperwork'. Such comments might show a fundamental lack of understanding of the role of the sister, as well as of what is meant by management, as was found in the studies of Williams (1969) and Runciman (1982). Looking again at Pembrey's study, let us see whether it is true that if a sister manages, she will not have patient or staff contact. The managing sister spent 17%

of her day working with patients, whereas the non-managing sister spent 22% of her day with patients. 'There!', you may say, 'all that managing does take sister away from the patients'. I agree that there is a 5% difference, or approximately 22 minutes out of a $7\frac{1}{2}$ hour shift, but not the 19% difference in time spent managing and not managing.

As this book is about learning in the work-place, let us now look at the sister in relation to the nurses in the ward as well as to the patients. If the amount of time the sister worked with patients is subdivided into the amount of time she worked with a patient alone or with a nurse *and* a patient, more light is shed on the matter (see Table 2.1). The managing sister spent 12% of her day working with patients and nurses, compared with 3% of the non-managing sister's day. While the managing sister spent 5% of her day working alone with patients, the non-managing sister spent 19% of her day in this way.

Earlier in the chapter, Marson (1982) highlighted the contribution that role-modelling can make to learning. The sister who works alone caring for patients gets her own personal satisfaction. If she has planned the work of the nursing team so that she can work with a nurse while giving care, the opportunity for teaching will be there. By the way she talks to the patient she is modelling attitudes; by the way in which she carries out nursing care she is demonstrating skills and techniques. Depending on the needs and abilities of the nursing team, she may be working with a learner in her first clinical experience, or with a staff nurse to demonstrate a complex nursing procedure. All are ways of learning and working at the same time. As mentioned in the introduction, sisters are often heard to say, 'I haven't time to teach', but by working with the nurse, the sister *is* teaching at the same time as getting the work done!

In another research study (Ogier, 1982), sisters were audiorecorded while they worked. Those sisters who were rated most highly by nurse learners spent only half of their time on duty interacting with anyone! Of the time they were interacting, nearly half was spent with nurse learners. When the sister–learner interactions were analysed, the content of the interactions shed more light on teaching/learning while-you-work, as demonstrated in the following examples.

1. *Sister*: 'Mary (*student nurse*), can you come here and check this controlled drug with me? Mrs Gavey last had pethidine at 6 a.m.; it is now 10 a.m., so she can have more.' Sister and nurse can be heard preparing syringes, counting the stock

and administering the drug to Mrs Gavey. Following the documentation, they clear up and go their separate ways.

2. *Sister*: 'Mary (*student nurse*), can you check this controlled drug with me? As you heard at the report, Mrs Gavey had a cholecystectomy yesterday afternoon. She last had pethidine 75 mg at 6 a.m.; it is now 10 a.m., and the physiotherapist is due to see her at about 10.30 a.m. If we give her more pethidine now, it will be working by the time the physiotherapist comes to help Mrs Gavey with her deep-breathing exercises.' While sister is talking, the injection is being prepared, and the sound of syringes being unwrapped and drug cupboards being unlocked can be heard. They administer the drug and sign the documentation, and, while clearing up, sister asks Mary, 'Are you getting on all right?'

Exercises

Imagine you are Mary; list what information was imparted in the interaction described in Example 1, and then do the same for Example 2. Which interaction conveys the most information?

Giving the drug took the same length of time in each example, but in the second one, sister was sharing her decision-making process – why the pethidine was being given – with the nurse. The effect on Mrs Gavey was the same in both cases, but in the second case, Mary gained an insight into the planning of pain-free recovery to aid the prevention of complications.

If Mary was asked what she had been taught, she would probably reply that it had been a busy morning and that she had been taught nothing! (see also Fretwell, 1982). If she was asked about postoperative analgesia and the prevention of complications, she would probably be able to recall the incident with Mrs Gavey. She has learnt through experience, which was triggered by sister's full explanation while they worked *together*.

HINTS FOR PRACTICE

- *Plan the work so as to enjoy patient care*, while working with a member of the nursing team, who can be supervised and taught by sharing knowledge and skills as well as by modelling caring, professional attitudes.

● *Talk through decision-making,* so that the inexperienced nurse can begin to identify the rationale for various nursing prescriptions and actions.

Exercise

Stop for a few minutes and think about how you manage your working day. Is it management by crisis, dashing from one urgent job to the next? Or do you manage in the sense that you assess, plan, implement and evaluate? Or are you managing in the sense that you contrive to get by with difficulty?

There are many aspects of patient care that are beyond the control of a nurse, some of which have been mentioned earlier. Lelean (1973) highlights the fact that sisters are frequently interrupted in their work, and that communication with nurses is of short duration; in her study, 85% of the informal communication of the sister with the ward nursing team lasted for less than one minute. It is essential to minimise interruptions in order to manage effectively, since after each interruption it takes time to get back to the original activity (Adair, 1987).

Exercise

Choose a 10-minute period in the day when the clinical area is at its quietest, and tell all your staff that it is *your* 10 minutes of thinking/planning time. At first you may find that you can get little done in that short interval, but if you unwind and take stock of the nursing activities for which you are accountable, you will have made a start. You may think that 10 minutes is not worth while, but if you are not in the habit of having time to manage, it is unrealistic to expect you or your staff to cope with longer periods.

Adair goes on to say that to learn to manage interruptions takes resolve and practice.

THE SISTER AS LEADER OF THE NURSING TEAM

The author carried out a study in an attempt to identify the attributes of ward sisters who were consistently identified by nurse learners as 'being good for learning' or just 'good' (Ogier, 1982). She felt that if specific attributes could be identified, other sisters and staff nurses could then be helped to develop the appropriate behaviours. The leadership style of the ward sisters was measured, in order to see whether the way in which they led their nursing teams affected the learning available in the clinical area, by asking them to complete Fleishman's Leadership Opinion Questionnaire (LOQ; Fleishman, 1969). The LOQ provides two measures of the leader's behaviour towards subordinates, consideration and structure.

Consideration reflects the extent to which an individual is likely to have job relationships with his subordinates characterised by mutual trust, respect for their ideas, consideration for their feelings and a certain warmth between himself and them. A high score is indicative of a climate of good rapport and two-way communication. A low score indicates that the individual is likely to be more impersonal in his relationships with group members.

Structure reflects the extent to which an individual is likely to define his own role and those of his subordinates towards goal attainment. A high score on this dimension characterises an individual who plays an active role in directing group activities through planning, communicating information, scheduling, criticising, trying out new ideas, and so forth. A low score characterises individuals who are likely to be relatively inactive in these ways.

The study, and subsequent use of the LOQ with over 400 ward sisters in the UK, showed that while it was always best to have high levels of consideration (that is, good rapport and two-way communication with subordinates), the optimum level of structure varied with the type of ward or department and with whether the subordinates were experienced nurses or nurse learners. In general medical and surgical wards with two or three trained nurses and the remainder of the team being unqualified nurses, a moderate degree of structure was required, with scores of 45–50 (maximum score possible 80). In specialist wards, such as neurosurgery or coronary care, where life-threatening situations occurred frequently, or where the staff were unfamiliar with the work, scores of up to 60 for structure (a high level) were tolerated by subordinates. This makes sense in the light of the definition of structure. In areas such as care of the elderly, where the work was often very heavy but predictable and where there was a high level of long-established staff, lower levels of structure, 35–40, were appropriate.

Where a sister has an inappropriate level of structure for the work and the calibre of the staff, either too organised, or not directive enough, junior nurses become unhappy. They either feel so directed that they are like automatons doing the bidding of the leader, or they lack direction and drift along in a disorganised manner. Neither state is 'good' for the junior nurse, who will eventually become either unthinking and unquestioning, where there is too much structure, or disorganised, where there is too little direction. Remember, as well as the direct effect on the subordinate of the sister's leadership style, the sister is teaching by being a very powerful role model. The over-organising sister is as likely to have staff nurses develop like her as is the disorganised sister. Ogier and Barnett (1986), in a tiny study of only 15 sisters and their staff nurses, were able to measure the role-modelling effect in 13 of the 15 sisters, using the LOQ for sister and staff nurses. The newly appointed staff nurse's LOQ score bore little resemblance to the score of the sister with whom she was working; staff nurses who had been in post with sister for a year had LOQ scores close to those of sister, while staff nurses who had been in post for 18 months had LOQ scores that were virtually identical with those of the sister.

The learners in the clinical areas completed a questionnaire about the sister and the ward – the Learners Perception of Ward Climate (LPWC). The questionnaire, developed for the study, was composed of 27 statements. During developmental testing of the questionnaire, it became apparent from the learners' point of view that 11 questions differentiated between the 'ideal' sisters and those not so. The 'ideal' sisters had a high level of consideration and a level of structure appropriate to the nature of the work as measured by the LOQ. The 'ideal' sisters were able to adapt their style of leadership and behaviour to suit the needs of student nurses, whether the latter were gaining experience in their first clinical allocation or were about to qualify and become staff nurses.

Many of the sisters were neither highly nor lowly rated. On inspection of the rating of these 'middle' sisters, the LPWC scores for senior and junior learners were analysed. The majority of the middle group of sisters fell into one of two categories: 'the mother hen' or 'the autocrat'. The 'mother hen' type of sister cared for her brood of learners by careful explanation and direction, watching over their every move. Junior learners thrived in this protective atmosphere, rating sister highly. Learners who were about to qualify were anxious to 'stretch their wings' and to begin to make decisions and plan their own work, were stifled and frustrated and rated sister low. The autocratic sisters were just the opposite: senior learners were happy to work within their delegated sphere, but new learners felt very unsupported and lost and fearful of doing wrong.

Jacka and Lewin (1987) asked students to rate the sister for approachability on a 1–10 point scale, 1 being very unapproachable and 10 very approachable. The mean for all sisters was 7.6, but individual sisters were rated from 10 to 1.3. Staff nurses were rated as more approachable.

These findings closely relate to the management of the clinical area, in that accurate assessment of the situation – that is, the nursing team's abilities and needs as well as the patients' needs – is essential if skilful planning is to take place, so that utilisation of the full potential of the team, to the benefit of the patient, can occur, and so that the team can learn and grow from each experience. The 'ideal' sisters, from the learners' perspective, were also identified as 'good' managers and care-givers, being highly rated by their peers, seniors and medical staff, as well as by patients and relatives.

HINTS FOR PRACTICE

- *Know your own strengths and weaknesses.* Build on your strengths, compensate for or reduce your weaknesses.
- *Assess the needs and abilities of the nursing team.*
- *Be sufficiently directive,* so that staff know where they are going.
- *Have clear goals that you expect to be achieved.* Lelean (1973) looked at nursing communication and report time. Her findings clearly show that nursing instructions were ambiguous. Statements such as 'can mobilise' and 'encourage fluids' were interpreted in different ways by each member of the nursing team, often with a wide variety of meaning.

- *Ensure that the staff understand the goals and how they are to be met.*
- *Be approachable,* so that staff can clarify issues rather than blunder on, making mistakes and learning bad habits from each other.
- *Provide motivation; make sure you are rewarding good work with positive consequences.* Jim is a capable staff nurse, so do you always allocate him to the illest patients, with the least experienced staff, because he will always cope, while allocating Jane, who is less able, to the fitter patients, with the support of a third year student? Think! Is that rewarding good work, and how long will Jim carry on taking the greater burden?
- *Give feedback on performance.* Do you really know how you perform, or do you think you must be doing all right because no one has complained? As leader, do not leave your team wondering!

Several of these ideas will be explored in more detail in Chapter 4, but are included here to provide some thoughts before moving on.

The work environment needs to be planned and the nursing team to be led with understanding, so that all participants may grow and develop, especially in a constantly changing organisation like the National Health Service. International Encounter (1987) reported that:

'Strong leaders are necessary, particularly for organisations that must undergo significant change. Not just good managers or executors but people who are value driven. Leaders who know how to mobilize the will of others, leaders who provide motivation and direction, leaders who feel strongly about issues, leaders who are thinkers as well as doers.'

Some of the studies which specifically look at learning and teaching in the clinical area will be considered in the next section.

THE SISTER AS TEACHER

At the start of her study, Fretwell (1982) reviewed the available literature about the ward sister as teacher, and she found that earlier work studies revealed that sisters spend little time in teaching. Lelean (1973) found that sisters spend less than − 2% of their time on duty communicating with junior nurses, and Lamond (1974) reported that the sister was not the most important teacher – in the transmission of technical skills anyone with sufficient skills and knowledge would teach the nurses. Jacka and Lewin (1987) found that, on average, students spent half their time on duty working on their own, and a few students spent as much as three quarters of their time working alone, rather than being supervised or paired with a trained nurse.

Fretwell decided to look at the recipients of teaching, the student nurses, rather than the teachers. The first part of her study was exploratory:

- to rank and identify wards with 'good' and 'less good' learning environments, by using the opinions of learners;
- to describe the characteristics of wards identified as 'good' learning environments;
- to describe the sisters' perceptions of their management and teaching roles.

She also explored students' perceptions of themselves as learners or workers. She found that learners who were involved in almost two thirds of basic nursing activities were fulfilling the worker role where no teaching or learning took place. Even nurses in their first ward experience felt competent in many basic tasks and did not feel the need for further practice. However, students did feel that they were learners when doing technical nursing, and felt that they needed supervision and practice. Fretwell (1980a) writes:

> 'It seems clear that what the learner gains from her environment depends on how she conceptualises her work and the way she has categorised previous experience. If the patient is seen as a work object on whom a series of easy routine jobs are done, basic care is reduced to monotony so that current experiences add little to the nurse's existing knowledge.'

The importance that sisters attached to teaching varied with their individual values and beliefs about nursing and nurse training (Marson, 1982). Sisters in 'acute' wards tended to rate technical nursing competence as being the most important. Sisters in long-term care wards rated changing attitudes as most important. Marson said that higher-level skills inherent in management of patient care, interpersonal skills and problem-solving and decison-making skills were rarely mentioned.

Fretwell, in her 1982 study, found that there was a variety of teachers in the ward, but that no dominant group assumed the role of teacher; indeed, in some wards learners were estimated to do more teaching than the trained nurse! Where task allocation and rigid routine were practised in the wards, learning opportunities were low, learners' powers of discovery were curtailed and job performance became automatic – 'just routine'.

While Fretwell did not find the sister to be the dominant teacher, she does conclude in her study that the sister is the key person who controls the learning environment. She writes (1980b):

> 'An ideal learning environment is seen as one in which the educational needs of learners are met – it is created by the sister and other trained nurses working in the ward. It is anti-hierarchical and key features are teamwork, negotiation, good communications and availability of trained nurses during and when work is done.'

Marson (1982) also highlights the fact that sisters may be unaware of nurses' learning needs and see teaching as a didactic process – sitting nurse down and 'teaching her'. Marson suggests that learning in the work-place might be enhanced by emphasis being shifted away from teaching as a didactic activity, and being placed on learning as personal development. Responsibility should be placed squarely on the learners, with sisters seeing themselves as helping learners to learn, rather than as teaching them, i.e. sisters acting as facilitators rather than teachers. Marson lists five main areas of competence for the trained nurse who may be considered 'good' at teaching:

1. *Professional qualities,* e.g. 'She kept good standards of nursing'.
2. *Managerial abilities,* e.g. 'The ward ran like clockwork'.
3. *Personality traits,* e.g. 'She was approachable and friendly'.
4. *Emphatic qualities,* e.g. 'She seemed to know how learners felt'.
5. *Teaching abilities,* e.g. 'He asked me questions to find out what I already knew; she explained medical terms in simple language'.

Similar qualities were perceived as important by nurses in Eire (McGowan, 1979).

However, the whole emphasis cannot be placed entirely upon the sisters, because, as mentioned at the beginning of Chapter 1, sisters do not function in a vacuum – rather, they have to work within the constraints of a vast, unwieldy organisation. When Fretwell (1985), building on her original study, undertook an action research project to assist sisters to become more able 'teachers' or facilitators of learning, she found that many organisational issues had to be dealt with in order to enable the sisters to develop the skills and attitudes needed to enhance learning.

A similar situation was found by Bryant (1985), who considered the role and preparation of the ward sister involved in nurse training. She found that the integration of theory and practice in the curriculum for students was hindered by a lack of .communication between teachers and ward sisters. Although sisters sought a 'partnership' with nurse teachers, it was often lacking. This contributed to a lack of clarity of the role of sister as a teacher. The majority of the 15 sisters studied felt ill-prepared for their teaching role, and had varied ideas on what was expected of them. Bryant was then able to build on her findings, as did Fretwell, and to develop a training programme for sisters, considering the relation of theory to practice and the role expectations of the ward sister. Jacka and Lewin (1987) reported that of 17 484 procedures and activities experienced by students throughout their training, and about which they had received instruction in school, 642 were reported to be items for which the school teaching did not precisely match ward practice, that is, 3.7% of all items.

Alexander (1982) was also concerned with integrating theory and practice in nursing. She carried out an educational experiment using a method of teaching that was intended to integrate theory and practice. In an exploratory study prior to the educational experiment, she found that student nurses reported a number of instances of disparity between theory and practice. She also found a very marked difference in the amount of ward teaching provided by ward staff and student nurses, when compared with that provided by teaching staff (the latter making a very small contribution) – a finding that is frequently supported by anecdotal accounts from sisters in various parts of the UK.

Some of Alexander's conclusions are that:

- student nurses need help in learning how to learn from their everyday work with patients;
- students need help to apply theory to practice and to use facts learned in the classroom in a variety of clinical experiences with individual patients.

This help needs to come from those who are trained to teach. Alexander writes:

'The giving of this help cannot be left in such a large measure to ward sisters, staff nurses and fellow students. Some of it always will be and indeed ought to be but is it right that this is done without giving these nurses any training either in teaching skills or in developing an awareness of how potent a force they are as role models in transmitting not only techniques of nursing but their own values as to the way nursing is?'

Alexander's findings echo Marson's (1982) results, in which three components were identified from the learners' perspective of ward teaching. These were:

- the power of the role model presented to the learner;
- skill in forming and managing interpersonal relationships;
- the art of being a good communicator.

Marson says that nurses perceive effective 'teachers' as caring, competent nurses and skilled team leaders. These 'teacher' nurses are sensitive to learners' needs, and make efforts to motivate and involve learners, providing them with feedback when needed: 'Teacher nurses are skilled in interpersonal relationships and demonstrate a personal value system of care and concern for others'.

HINTS FOR PRACTICE

- *Are you competent and up to date?* Now, don't take offence; the busier you are, the quicker time passes, so check up on when you last updated your knowledge, reviewed your skills and reflected upon your attitudes.
- *Are you hanging on to long-cherished routines, regardless of the needs of the individual patient and research evidence?* Does everyone have to be bathed by 10 a.m. or, at the very latest, before lunch? Are your patients made worse by prolonged preoperative fasting? (Hamilton-Smith, 1972; replicated by Thomas, 1987).
- *What kind of role model are you?* Look back over what you have just read in this chapter. Are you a managing leader, with a clear idea of the educational needs of the nursing team and/or colleagues, or are you managing in the sense that you are getting by or coping, rather than being in control. Even if you are not the nurse in charge, you will have some management and leadership responsibilities towards patients and other members of the nursing team.
- *Are you a communicator?* Do you tell or do you listen?
- *Do you know what the learners are taught in the classroom in relation to your area?* If you don't know, why don't you know? Have you ever asked or been asked to talk about *your* work in the classroom? Time spent in the classroom, perhaps one hour, will be more than saved by the learners coming with a clear

perception of what is entailed, and by not having to learn one thing for the 'school' and one for the ward (Bendall, 1972; Hunt, 1974; Gott, 1984).

• *Have you completed a teaching and assessing course for clinical staff?* Have you ever asked to do one? In England the ENB course no. 998 is designed for nurses in the clinical area. What have you in your area to help you?

• *What values do you have about nursing and the care of the individual?* Are your values demonstrated in your attitudes and behaviours? Be honest with yourself.

• *Do you radiate enthusiasm and exhibit satisfaction when a job is well done?*

THE SISTER AS CREATOR OF THE LEARNING CLIMATE

Orton (1981) opens her monograph with the following quotation from a student nurse:

> 'Everyone who came on the ward was immediately aware of the happy atmosphere which influenced all our relationships with staff and patients. Everyone was willing to teach us and we learnt a fantastic amount during our time there.'

The importance of the 'atmosphere' in the clinical area, and of the role of the ward sister in creating that atmosphere, has been referred to in earlier parts of this chapter and considered by earlier writers, such as Perry (1978):

> '. . . if the ward sister is a good leader each member of the team is given the satisfaction of making the maximum contribution to patient care in accordance with her particular talents, knowledge, skills and experience; thus a happy atmosphere is engendered. This is essential to the well being of both patients and staff but, in addition, it encourages learning. Furthermore, there is order in a well managed ward. Each member of the team knows what to do and has the necessary resources available to do it.'

Jacka and Lewin (1987) asked students to list those aspects of their present ward that:

• helped them most;
• hindered their learning.

They found that the aspect that helped most was ward atmosphere, and the factor that hindered learning was ward 'tempo' and workload; however, atmosphere was the second most inhibiting factor. Sisters also found that a good atmosphere helped their teaching role, rating it third in importance of those aspects that were most helpful. However, their teaching role was hardly affected by poor atmosphere.

The research of Pembrey (1980) into the management abilities of the ward sister and the findings of Ogier (1982) about the sister's leadership style go to support the writings of Perry that the ability of the sister to utilise and develop her staff is crucial for all concerned. Orton's study (1981) set out to determine whether the ward learning climate existed as a measurable reality for student nurses. Let us look at some of the findings.

Orton concludes that there is a definite measurable property of the ward environment. In order to identify the dimensions of a ward learning climate, student nurses completed questionnaires that had been designed for this study. Analysis of the questionnaires revealed two aspects: 'ward sister recognition of student nurse needs' and 'ward sister's teaching commitment'. Of 12 wards studied, three were highly rated. Orton called these 'high student orientation (referred to as 'high' wards); three wards were at the other extreme – 'low student orientation' (referred to as 'low' wards). The remaining wards fell between the two extremes. Orton writes:

> 'The hallmark of a high student orientation ward was the combination of teamwork, consultation and ward sister awareness of the needs of the subordinates. Not only did students see their own physical and emotional needs amply met but also those of the patients.'

The ward sisters' self-reports also supported the students' opinions, with Orton's work reinforcing Pembrey's, Ogier's, Marson's and Fretwell's studies discussed earlier. Facilitating learning cannot be divorced from competent management and humane leadership. A closer look at the responses to some of the questions on Orton's student nurse questionnaire shows that they differentiated between high student-orientated sisters and low student-orientated sisters, as well as showing how they related to responses in other studies.

● 'All staff on the ward, from the sister to the newest recruit feel part of the ward team': in the high wards 90% of the students agreed with this statement, while in the low wards 66% of students disagreed.

● 'The ward sister regards the student nurse as a worker rather than as a learner': in the high wards 82% of students disagreed, while in the low wards 65% agreed.

● 'I did not feel I was treated as an individual, but merely as just another learner': in high wards 79% of the students disagreed, but in the low wards 70% agreed.

The results of these three questions from Orton's study are similar to findings of the author's own study. Student nurses in Ogier's study said spontaneously that they wanted to work where they felt they were part of a team, whereas Orton asked the specific question of her students. Whichever way the information is gathered, the same emphasis on the importance of the sister and her ability as leader and manager to create an environment where it is safe to learn keeps recurring. King (1986) wrote:

> 'A climate that is free from threat without being free from challenge is essential for learning. When learners have a feeling of acceptance and belonging, they tend to set goals. . . Learners have a need for recognition by peers and teachers.'

Like Orton, the author was also interested in whether students saw themselves as learners or workers, since it was felt that this might affect their uptake of available learning opportunities. Prior to their first clinical allocation, 44 student nurses felt like a learner for 96% of the time, and also like a worker for 62% of the time. However, at the end of their first allocation, these same students felt like learners for 64% of the time and workers for 80%! Other groups of students at the end of their second and third years of training felt much more like workers than learners; 95 and 100% respectively as workers, and 28 and 34% as learners.

These findings throw light on how student nurses perceive themselves in the clinical area, which has also been discussed in relation to Fretwell's study earlier in this chapter.

The relationship between nurse learners' perceptions and the activities of the ward sister is further highlighted by the third example drawn from Orton's questionnaire: 'I do not feel I was treated as an individual but merely as just another learner'.

As described earlier in the section on leadership and the ward sister, a questionnaire was developed in order to differentiate between ward sisters who were 'ideal' for nurse learners and those who were not. Eleven key questions were identified, which would separate the ideal from the non-ideal sister. Two of the key questions on the Learners Perception of Ward Climate (LPWC) are:

- 'Sister is interested in me';
- 'Sister is helpful to me'.

The statements were derived from responses given by nurses in training to the request to describe helpful instances, or 'good' things, and the opposite, in their last ward experience. When developing the questionnaire, student nurses were asked what was meant by 'Sister is interested in me', and how it differed from 'Sister is helpful to me'. Their replies indicated that they appreciate the sister who knows them as a person. For example, Avril Le Pelley is in her second year of training. This is her second medical ward experience, and she hopes to extend her skills in caring for patients with a poor prognosis and to learn more about neurological disorders, rather than just be a student nurse in the ward for 8 or 12 weeks. 'Sister is helpful to me' appeared to be more impersonal, in that sister would be willing to assist any nurse.

Seventy per cent of the students involved in testing the LPWC replied that the 'ideal' sister was always or often interested in them, and 83% said she was always or often helpful to them, while 82% found that the 'non-ideal' sister was never interested in them, and 88% said the 'non-ideal' sister was never helpful to them.

These results are very similar to Marson's and Orton's findings, supporting the importance of the ward climate for patient and staff well-being. Possibly the single most influential person in setting the tone of the climate is the ward sister.

The importance of the ward sister in creating a climate of care was acknowledged in the Skill Mix Report (1986), where it states that:

> 'Our overwhelming impression is that the quality and cost effectiveness of care depended crucially on the leader of the ward nursing team. In long stay areas in particular, it was the sister or charge nurse who was the determining influence on the style and pattern of care, other personnel playing a less central role.'

For as Orton concludes:

> 'What is now certain is that the encouragement and development of 'good' learning climates would bring about improvements for all those involved in ward life and that the benefits could be measured not only in economic terms but also by the increase in human happiness and well-being.'

Lindop (1987), looking at the factors affecting wastage of nurses in training, says that the need for a deeper understanding of the personal reactions of nurses in training, as well as of stressors and how these affect such nurses, is clearly indicated. This is not a new concept and much has been written about stress and nursing. Wilson (1974) wrote that nurses will experience stress in their training, but what he considers to be important is not that learners are protected from stress, but rather that they should be supported and grow through a stressful experience:

> 'The care which a nurse learner receives is an important source of her own care of others. One of the ripest fruits of education is to develop in a student an open attitude to people and events as they happen.'

It is apparent from some of the work considered earlier in this book that training and socialisation have often resulted in qualified nurses becoming closed, unquestioning individuals, maybe for their self-protection (Menzies, 1970). Some nurses will need help and support in order to become open, caring individuals. To conclude with a quotation from an examination paper (therefore no attribution is possible): 'Minds are like parachutes – they work better when they are open!'

HINTS FOR PRACTICE

● When completing previous exercises, you will have made lists of learning opportunities in the clinical area and compared these with student nurses' perception of the learning available to them. If you did not do this then, do so now. Are you in touch with what are perceived to be the needs of your colleagues, peers and juniors? Time that is given to considering the needs of the nursing team will reap great dividends for patient care, as morale rises and individuals become more sensitive to themselves and others. This is not a new idea – it is well documented as the 'Hawthorne effect', first described in 1939 (Roethlisberger and Dickson, 1939). This states that paying attention to people at work improves their performance.

The original study was done at the Hawthorne works of the Western Electric Company in California, where the management wanted better productivity, and tried to achieve this by improving or altering working conditions, such as upgrading the lighting and changing the shifts. Everything they did increased productivity, even when this included returning to the original working conditions. The conclusion is that changing external working conditions does not affect performance as much as the workers' perception that someone is interested in *them* and their work.

The knowledge of the Hawthorne effect has been used in several industries to improve performance, with beneficial results, yet little notice is taken of NHS employees, who may be required to function like unquestioning drones. Indeed, Rowbottom et al (1973) wrote:

'Ultimately it has to be accepted that a hospital is for treating patients not employing staff in satisfying conditions.'

Well, you cannot revolutionise the entire NHS, but what you can do is to ensure that your colleagues, peers and juniors feel needed and valued, however small their contribution.

- *Know the staff as individuals,* not just as a newly qualified staff nurse or yet another first ward student nurse.
- Having regard to what you have just read in this chapter, make sure that:
- *the goals you set yourself and others are explicit, achievable and easily understood;*
- *you give feedback on performance;*
- *you are approachable;*
- *you let your caring enthusiasm shine through;* remember that you are a role model.

Exercise

Now list some specific tips or pointers for yourself. Try to be precise and give yourself a time limit in which to review your progress. You may want to share the tips with a colleague you can trust, so that you have a mentor on whom to try out ideas and who will give you support.

'Efficiency, it has been said, is doing things right, while effectiveness is doing the right things.' (Adair, 1987)

May you be both efficient *and* effective.

References

Adair J (1987) *How to Manage Your Time.* Surrey: Talbot Adair/McGraw Hill.
Alexander M F (1982) Integrating theory and practice in nursing – 1 and 2. *Nursing Times,* Occasional Papers, **78**(17): 65–68; **78**(18): 69–71.
Bendall E (1972) *So You Passed Nurse.* RCN Research Series. London: Royal College of Nursing.
Bryant R J (1985) *The Role and Preparation of the Ward Sister Involved in Nurse Training.* MSc dissertation, Dept of Educational Studies, University of Surrey.

Buccheri R C (1986) Nursing supervision: a new look at an old role. *Nursing Administration Quarterly*, **11**(1): 11–25.

Child D (1986) *Psychology and the Teacher*, 4th edn. London: Holt Education.

Farnish E G S (1983) *Ward Sister Preparation. A Survey of Three Districts.* London: Nursing Education Research Unit, King's College, University of London.

Fleishman E A (1969) *Manual for Leadership Opinion Questionnaire.* Chicago: Science Research Associates Inc.

Fretwell J E (1980a) Hospital ward routine – friend or foe? *Journal of Advanced Nursing*, **5**: 625–636.

Fretwell J E (1980b) An inquiry into the ward learning environment. *Nursing Times*, Occasional Paper, **76**(16): 69–75.

Fretwell J E (1982) *Ward Teaching and Learning: Sister and the Learning Environment.* RCN Research Series. London: Royal College of Nursing.

Fretwell J E (1985) *Freedom to Change. The creation of a Ward Learning Environment.* RCN Research Series. London: Royal College of Nursing.

Gott M (1984) *Learning Nursing. A Study of the Effectiveness and Relevance of Teaching Provided During Student Nurse Introductory Course.* RCN Research Series. London: Royal College of Nursing.

Hall B A, von Endt L and Parker G (1981) A framework for measuring satisfaction of nursing staff. *Nursing Leadership*, **4**(4): 29–33.

Hamilton-Smith S (1972) *Nil by Mouth.* RCN Research Series. London: Royal College of Nursing.

Hunt J (1974) *The Teaching and Practice of Surgical Dressings in Three Hospitals.* London: Royal College of Nursing.

International Encounter (1987) *Leadership in Nursing for Health for All. A Challenge and Strategy for Action.* Report on Conference, 'An International Encounter on Leadership in Nursing for Health for All', Tokyo, Japan, 7–11 April 1986. Geneva: World Health Organisation.

Jacka K and Lewin D (1987) *The Clinical Learning of Student Nurses.* NERU Report No. 6. London: Nursing Education Research Unit, Kings College, University of London.

James D E (1970) *Introduction to Psychology.* London: Panther Science.

Jarvis P (1983) *Professional Education.* London: Croom Helm.

King I M (1986) *Curriculum and Instruction in Nursing. Concepts and Process.* Norwalk, Connecticut: Appleton-Century-Crofts.

Knowles M (1984) *The Adult Learner: A Neglected Species.* Houston: Gulf Publishing Co.

Lamond N (1974) *Becoming a Nurse. The Registered Nurse's View of General Student Nurse Education.* RCN Research Series. London: Royal College of Nursing.

Lathlean J (ed.) (1988) *Research in Action: Developing the Role of the Ward Sister.* London: King's Fund Centre.

Lathlean J, Smith G and Bradley S (1986) *Post-Registration Development Schemes Evaluation.* NERU Report No. 4. London: Nursing Education Research Unit, King's College, University of London.

Layton M M Sr (1969) How instructors' attitudes affect students. *Nursing Outlook*, **17**(1): 20–27.

Lelean S R (1973) *Ready for Report Nurse? A Study in Nursing Communication in Hospital Wards.* RCN Research Series. London: Royal College of Nursing.

Lindop E (1987) Factors associated with student and pupil nurse wastage. *Journal of Advanced Nursing*, **12**(6): 751–756.

Marson S N (1982) Ward sister – teacher or facilitator? An investigation into behavioural characteristics of effective ward teachers. *Journal of Advanced Nursing*, 7(4): 347–357.

Menzies I E P (1970) *Social Systems as a Defence Against Anxiety*. London: The Tavistock Institute of Human Relations.

McGowan J (1979) *Attitude Survey of Irish Nurses*. Dublin, Eire: Institute of Public Administration.

National Health Service Training Authority (1986) *Better Management, Better Health*. Bristol: NHSTA.

Ogier M E (1982) *An Ideal Sister? A Study of the Leadership Style and Verbal Interactions of Ward Sisters with Nurse Learners in General Hospitals*. RCN Research Series. London: Royal College of Nursing.

Ogier M E (1986) An 'ideal' sister – seven years on. *Nursing Times*, Occasional Papers, 82(2): 54–57.

Ogier M E and Barnett D E (1986) Sister/staff nurse and the nurse learner. *Nurse Education Today*, 6: 16–22.

Orton H D (1981) *Ward Learning Climate. A Study of the Role of the Ward Sister in Relation to Student Nurse Learning on the Ward*. RCN Research Series. London: Royal College of Nursing.

Pembrey S (1980) *The Ward Sister – Key to Nursing. A Study of the Organisation of Individualised Nursing*. RCN Research Series. London: Royal College of Nursing.

Perry E L (1978) *Ward Management and Teaching*. London: Baillière Tindall.

Quinn F M (1988) *The Principles and Practice of Nurse Education*. London: Croom Helm.

Redfern S J (1980) Hospital sisters: work attitudes, perceptions and wastage. *Journal of Advanced Nursing*, 5: 451–466.

Reid N G (1985) *Wards in Chancery? Nurse Training in the Clinical Area*. RCN Research Series. London: Royal College of Nursing.

Revans R W (1961) *The Measurement of Supervisory Attitudes*. Manchester: Manchester Statistical Society.

Roethlisberger F J and Dickson W J (1939) *Management and the Worker*. Boston: Harvard University Press.

Rowbottom R, Balle J, Cang S, Dixon M, Jacques E, Packwood T and Tolliday H (1973) *Hospital Organisation*. London: Heinemann.

Runciman P (1982) Ward sisters: their problems at work – 1 and 2. *Nursing Times*, Occasional Papers, 78(36): 141–143; 78(37): 145–147.

Skill Mix Report (1986) *Mix and Match: A Review of Nursing Skill Mix*. Chairman: Miss Patsy Wright-Warren. London: DHSS.

Thomas E A (1987) Pre-operative fasting – a question of routine? *Nursing Times*, Occasional Papers, 83(7): 46–47.

van Hoozer H L, Bratton B D, Ostmoe P M, Weinholtz D, Craft M J, Gjerde C L and Albanese M A (1987) *The Teaching Process. Theory and Practice in Nursing*. Norwalk, Connecticut: Appleton-Century-Crofts.

Williams D (1969) The administrative contribution of the nursing sisters. *Public Administration*, 47: 307–328.

Wilson M (1974) The wider requirements of nursing education. In: *A Consultation on Wide Issues in Nursing Education* (conference papers). London: The Institute of Religion and Medicine.

3
Telling isn't Teaching, Teaching isn't Telling

The aim of this chapter is to relate some of the available theories to the research findings, to form a basis for effective and efficient learning while working.

Some of the research findings about the role of the ward sister, especially in connection with her ability to enhance the opportunity for learning and staff development in the clinical area, were considered in the previous chapter, and the latter finished with a wish to be both effective and efficient. While this is of prime importance for patients and clients, it is also vital to and inseparable from the development of the staff who provide this service. The present chapter will focus on a few ideas for encouraging staff to develop their clinical and professional expertise. This is not to suggest that such activities should replace 'off-the-job' education, but rather that staff should be helped to utilise the opportunities that are available in the clinical area. As we saw in earlier chapters, learning takes place best where it is needed and relates to practice (see Appendix I).

Nurses who have just completed an experience in a clinical area have been heard to cry, 'I wasn't *taught* anything', or sisters have been heard to say, 'I haven't time to teach'. What does the student or sister mean by teaching? As part of exploratory work at the beginning of the research study into the leadership style of the ward sister, the writer explored with groups of student nurses, staff nurses and sisters what they meant by teaching (Ogier, 1982). In the majority of instances, teaching was described as being the didactic situation of learners sitting down in front of a 'teacher' propounding a subject and writing on the blackboard – the 'talk and chalk' method. A few responses identified demonstration techniques, or aspects of care in the clinical area, and a few mentioned teaching while doing – the role model.

TELLING ISN'T TEACHING

Schmieding (1987) looked at the daily encounters of nurse managers with their subordinates, and at how those encounters could foster constructive participation in decision-making and problem-solving. When approached by a junior nurse with a problem, the majority of nurse managers did not open a dialogue on the matter; rather, they either dealt with the problem themselves, or told the nurse what to do, or asked an irrelevant question. By telling the nurse what to do, a valuable opportunity to explore ways of solving the problem with her was lost. Likewise, teaching is not just a matter of imparting information or telling; it is:

• creating an awareness for the need to learn;
• identifying learning opportunities;
• creating a climate in which it is 'safe' to learn;
• many other factors discussed earlier.

Effectiveness has been defined by Deane and Campbell (1985) as having an actual effect, such as the ability to bring about results, not merely a theoretical or potential effect. Lathlean (1988) describes how ward sisters, having been given the opportunity at a one-day colloquium of hearing about the research findings discussed in Chapter 2, went back to their work-place and, with their nurse manager and nurse teacher, each developed a project relevant to the needs of her work. They worked on their chosen project for between 6 and 18 months. Not all the sisters fulfilled their original aims, since some goals were set too high, but even those who did not complete the task which they had chosen described the exercise as helpful and identified learning, even by discovering what could not be done! Therefore, 'ordinary' clinical nurses can assimilate and use research findings for their own professional development. It is hoped that by the time you reach the end of this chapter, you will be reviewing your practice and setting yourself realistic goals to maintain and develop your professional effectiveness and competence.

Effective nurses know themselves, have a knowlege of theory and can use it to get the right things done at the right time (Douglass, 1980). As you read through the last chapter, you were asked to pause and consider various aspects of yourself and your performance; here we will build on and develop these ideas, so that you can develop or review your personal theory of practice, especially as it relates to your own learning and that of those with whom you work.

What is meant by a theory of practice? Argyris and Schön (1976) developed a theoretical framework for improving professional effectiveness. They propose that every individual has a set of theories, which explain, predict and control his or her behaviour. A theory of practice is made up of a person's interrelated theories of action. If I ask a community psychiatric nurse (CPN) how she assists the relatives of a very anxious client, the ways in which she describes her behaviours and decisions would be her 'theories of action'. However, if she was instead observed, how she actually behaved, negotiated, discussed, and so on, would be her 'theories in use'. It is well known that people do not always do what they say they do! In the nursing context, nurses saying or writing one thing and doing another has already been mentioned (Bendall, 1972; Lelean, 1973; Hunt, 1974; Alexander, 1982). To summarise, individuals have a set of theories which guide or control their behaviours:

- *theories of practice,* made up of interrelated
  - *theories of action,* which when put into action become
    - *theories in use.*

A theory of practice is individualised; it changes and develops as the person gains new knowledge, skills and abilities through various experiences.

Why bother with a theoretical framework? We began this chapter by being concerned with effectiveness, defined as the actual, rather than the theoretical? The framework provides a structure upon which to build competences related to teaching and learning in the clinical area. It may also help with thinking about the difficulty posed by people saying one thing but doing something else. Deane and Campbell (1985) write:

'A theory of practice cannot be static but must be responsive to new knowledge and experiences. Professional effectiveness and competence evolve as the nurse develops a personal theory of practice. Developing a theory of practice requires lifelong learning and accountability.'

Perhaps the starting point is where you and your colleagues are now, but since each one of you is an individual, it is impossible to begin in several places at once; therefore, a common denominator will be chosen, that of you as an adult. In Appendix I, Knowles' (1984) Andragogical Theory, the art and science of teaching adults, is discussed, and some of the assumptions are considered. Burnard (1987) writes that the principles of andragogy apply well to the development of nursing skills. Knowles sees the teacher of adults as a helper, and quotes Tough (1979) to support his view:

'Finally, the ideal helper is probably an open growing person not a closed, negative, static, defensive, fearful, or suspicious sort of person. He himself is frequently a learner and seeks growth and new experiences. He probably tends to be spontaneous and authentic, and to feel free to behave as a unique person rather than in some stereotyped way.'

As discussed earlier, the qualified nurse may well have been trained and socialised into becoming a conforming 'servant', providing care as directed by hospital procedures and policies. This is hardly preparing the nurse for the role of ideal helper. The principles of teaching and the conditions of learning depicted by Knowles may be helpful; by considering some of these, and by reviewing information covered in the previous chapters, an attempt is made here to relate relevant material to you, the reader, who is also an adult learner as well as a facilitator of other adults' learning.

The first condition for learning that Knowles outlines is that *the learners feel a need to learn*. The very fact that you are reading this book might justify the assumption that, at the very least, you are interested in learning. In the previous chapters you considered the learning opportunities available to you in the clinical area and faced the issue of whether your knowledge is up to date. As an ideal helper, how do you help your colleagues and peers to perceive the need to learn? Do you:

- point out how out of date and stuck in the mud they are?
- show them how much you know?
- threaten them with disciplinary action under the Code of Conduct?

Hardly; such actions are more likely to drive them away and/ or alienate them!

Exercise

Write down your ideas on how you may help a qualified nurse to become aware of the need to learn. At this stage, do not try to put the whole world to rights; choose one colleague, then list ideas for helping her to come to terms with the need to learn.

When one considers the research findings about a sister as a manager, the first step of the management cycle is to assess the situation. Assessment includes both patients' needs and the needs and abilities of the staff. Assessment of learning needs is one of the first principles of teaching identified by Knowles (1984). Knowles suggests that the teacher, having first identified the student's potential for self-fulfilment, helps her to identify hopes and goals for development. The teacher then assists the student to look at the gap between where she is and where she hopes to progress to.

You have earlier made a list of learning opportunities in your area, and it was suggested that you checked your list with your colleagues. That may well have been the first step in identifying not only what could be learnt, but also what learning is desirable. The exercise may have provided the impetus for helping peers and juniors to think about learning while working, thereby breaking the cycle of 'it's only routine'. Even if peers and juniors do not agree with you, at least the process towards further development has begun. The first step may be the hardest, especially for the nurse who has been qualified for ten or more years and who has received no further and continuing education since qualification.

Identifying the need to learn may be painful and, as looked at earlier (Cox, 1984), learning may be uncomfortable. The more that is learnt, the more there seems to be to learn! Thus, it is important that the assessment of learning needs and the actual learning take place in an environment which is supportive and conducive to learning (Orton, 1981; Ogier, 1982, 1986; Fretwell, 1985; see also Chapter 2).

The importance of the learning environment relates to the second condition for learning described by Knowles (1984). This is characterised by *mutual trust, respect* and *mutual helpfulness.* Indeed, these are the very characteristics which were identified in the research studies that were discussed earlier.

Knowles also emphasises the importance of *freedom of expression* and *acceptance of differences.* When a nurse approaches you with a nursing problem, do you always jump in with the answer or deal with the matter, rather than ask the nurse how she thinks the problem could be resolved (Schmieding, 1987)? Indeed, it may turn out not to be a problem, or what the nurse was asking may be a 'cover' to approach you for another reason. Opportunities for developing a colleague may easily be lost if your style of management and leadership is such as to inhibit the free exchange of ideas and questions. Shortage of time is often blamed: 'It's quicker to do it myself'. So might it be at the time, but then the nurse does not learn how to solve that problem, whether it is how to arrange a domiciliary visit for a patient who is about to be discharged, or how to order a particular drug. When the same problem recurs, the nurse will have to come back to you; you will do it again because it is quicker, and so on. Is it really quicker? You are spending your time doing what the nurse could or should be doing for her own development and satisfaction. You do not have the time to manage, and the nurse gets locked into a routine of daily chores, referring anything out of the ordinary to you and thereby becoming stifled. Thus, she stops developing professionally, and you become frustrated because you are unable to fulfil your proper role as manager and leader. The next time that a nurse approaches you with a problem, do not rush to solve it – rather, explore the nurse's reaction to the problem. She may have a better solution, but have been trained to follow the 'book' and conform. So be approachable, stop, think and listen before rushing in, so that you can gain from those around you and they can gain from your support and guidance (Porritt, 1984).

By encouraging the nurse to explore her own responses to the problem that she has posed, you will also help her to become aware of any deficiency in her knowledge or skills, without having to allude to them point-blank. If a nurse is aware of her deficiency, she is more likely to make learning goals to overcome it, and if she sets the goals, perhaps with guidance and support from you, she is far more likely to work to achieve them, rather than having goals or objectives imposed upon her. Knowles outlines similar conditions of learning: *learners perceive the goals of a learning experience to be their own goals*, and *learners accept a share of responsibility for the learning experience and, therefore, have a commitment to it.*

How much support and guidance the nurse needs will depend on her level of competence and commitment, which can be ascertained by the first step of the management cycle – assessment. Some health authorities have a system of staff appraisal, which is carried out at regular intervals by the individual's immediate superior. However, there are many instances where there is no formal appraisal system. Many sisters suppose that they must be performing well '. . . because someone soon tells you if you get it wrong, so while you hear nothing you must be doing all right'. Suppose that one of these sisters who has had no feedback on her own performance complains about the shortcomings of a particular staff nurse.

When asked whether discussing the difficulties with the staff nurse has made any difference, the sister looks amazed and replies that she has not discussed matters with the nurse, '. . . after all, she should know it is wrong!' Should she? Is the staff nurse in the same situation as the sister, presuming that since sister has not said anything, the staff nurse must be doing all right?

If there is no formal appraisal system in your work-place, make sure that you find time to talk to your juniors. Ask them how they think they are getting on, how they feel about their own progress and work in the unit or ward. *Listen* to their needs: you may find that your listening ability should be developed. Reddy (1987) has written a practical textbook for managers, with a view to helping them to listen more effectively and to respond in a constructive manner, while Porritt (1984) writes on communication specifically for nurses providing a very readable account with useful guidelines.

Once you have formulated some idea of your juniors' needs and abilities, you can then help them to set goals and make plans for their own development. How much direction they will need will depend upon their developmental level. Blanchard et al (1987) describe four developmental levels and suggest the appropriate leadership style:

Level 1: Low competence, high commitment. A nurse gaining her first ward experience might be at this level, having little knowledge and expertise but being very enthusiastic. She will need to be directed and supervised with a degree of control, since a little knowledge with a lot of enthusiasm could be quite dangerous, and it is possible that her enthusiasm might lead her to undertake a task for which she is not yet competent.

Level 2: Some competence, low commitment. A second year student nurse, in the middle of her training, might be at Level 2 of the developmental stages, in that she should have some competence but may have low commitment, since the first burst of enthusiasm has passed and finals, with qualifying, seem a long way off. This student will need a coaching style of leadership, to provide a sense of purpose and direction with support.

Level 3: High competence, variable commitment. This might apply to a part-time staff nurse who has been in post some time but who has not received additional stimulation or education; she may, therefore, have a high level of competence but variable commitment. For this staff nurse, the leadership style will need to be supportive, giving praise for good work, listening to ideas and enabling her to utilise her competences.

Level 4: High competence, high commitment. This is the final level described by Blanchard et al, such as may be found in a senior staff nurse. This staff nurse will blossom and develop if a delegating style of leadership is used, allowing her the opportunity of making decisions in running the ward or department. Remember that delegation does not mean abdication of responsibility!

In order to obtain the best from the staff and to facilitate their growth, all four types of leadership may be used during a period on duty. By being aware of the abilities as well as the limitations of members of staff, the work can be completed safely, at the same time as furthering their growth. By seeking to use appropriate styles of leadership for each individual in the nursing team, the teacher's own growth takes place as she develops the skills of managing people. Staff who see that the leader identifies them as individuals, recognises their needs and nurtures their abilities will respond by greater commitment and motivation, and, from their feeding back of ideas and information, a dynamic, thriving nursing team will result. McCloskey and Molen (1987) reviewed 58 American research reports on nursing leadership; they conclude that there is an association between management style and situational factors, and that, therefore, the educational preparation and personality variables may differ between organisations. However, they suggest that the key is to develop appropriate knowledge and skill, and then to be astute and flexible in adapting to situations.

Thus far in this chapter, we have tried to convey the message that learning in the work-place is not just a matter of expert presentation of information; rather, it is enabling the individuals who make up the work-force to use their expertise, and be able to acknowledge their weaknesses in an atmosphere that is supportive and rewarding. This will benefit all concerned – patient, client, staff and yourself – let alone the organisation within which the work is carried out. Rogers and Lawrence (1987) report that individuals are more likely to contribute actively to their working environment and to remain in post if they perceive that they have an opportunity to develop their own particular interests and skills within the job.

While this may be encouraging and exciting, it is essential to address the issues of the need for support. Learning can be uncomfortable, because long-cherished ideas have to be discarded, but this necessary pruning produces healthier growth. At a time of shortages of resources and manpower, increasing the awareness of what ideally should be done, of the quality of care and of trying to raise standards may have a stressful effect upon the staff, leading to moral distress. Moral distress is a state in which a person makes a moral decision but is unable to carry it through. For example, the nurse planning the care of a recently paralysed paraplegic patient will not only be concerned about his physical condition, but will also plan time to enable the patient to explore the implications of his altered condition, since a positive outlook is crucial for rehabilitation. However, owing to manpower shortages, it is impossible to spend the necessary time in adequate, meaningful discussion. The nurse feels frustrated and upset, and valuable energy is lost as the nurse has to observe the patient struggling to come to terms with his disability. Wilkinson (1985) interviewed staff nurses who had experienced moral distress. The most common causes of distress were:

- the prolonging of life;
- performing unnecessary tests and treatments on the terminally ill;
- in situations of truth-telling.

Many nurses find themselves in similar situations, with ward sisters in the UK reporting the distress that they feel when they know that the needs of the patients are not being met (personal communication). The more that nurses' awareness is increased, the greater is the need for a supportive environment, if increased distress is not to occur.

Ward or unit support groups for the staff can help. Support groups for workers in mental health are well established, and are being introduced into the area of general nursing, particularly in specialist units such as oncology. Members of the groups recognise the need to support each other, express anxieties and air grievances in a non-threatening environment. In a group that accepts that people are all different and feel different, a worry shared can be explored and possibly solved, or at least acknowledged by others; this may prevent the worry from festering and growing out of all proportion.

In addition, there may be peer support groups. In a peer support group, people of similar role or status meet to share their joys and their worries, and to discuss their good ideas and difficulties, thus finding out that they are not alone. Try to make a determined effort, each month or more frequently if

necessary, to arrange time when as many of your ﹖
can come together, not for a report or an update,
of finding out how each individual is progressii
It will be a time of learning – learning that you
Sisters may say, ' . . . but we have no time to co
care, let alone have staff meetings'. Time spent
supportive environment, perhaps for just 15 minutes, will be
more than recouped by renewed energies and the increased
well-being of the staff, since tensions can be defused and
misunderstandings cleared up. Moral distress can inhibit
adequate functioning, affect patient care and retard development
of the person concerned (Wilkinson, 1985). If you are concerned
that the meeting may just end up as a big moan, or get out of
hand, talk to a colleague who is already running such meetings.
Tschudin (1987) has some helpful advice about support groups
and the need for nurse support.

HINTS FOR PRACTICE

- *There is more to teaching than telling.*
- *Allow subordinates to think through problems,* help them to learn
and develop via problem-solving and decision-making (Jones,
1988).
- *Help staff to feel the need to learn and identify the goals they
wish to achieve* (Knowles, 1984).
- *Identify learning opportunities and help staff to be more sensitive
to learning by experience* (Orton, 1981; Fretwell, 1982, 1985; Ogier,
1982, 1986; Jacka and Lewin, 1987).
- In order to be effective as teacher and leader, *have a framework
within which to work* (Deane and Campbell, 1985).
- *Identify your own theory of practice,* i.e. what values, ideas,
and beliefs control the way in which you behave (Argyris and
Schön, 1976).
- *Do you really act in the ways in which you say or think you do?*
- One theory of practice is that the nurse is an adult learner.
As adult learners, you and your colleagues, peers and juniors
will be more inclined to learn if you *own* the need for
learning, and participate in setting and achieving goals. *Active
participation in the learning situations promotes learning.*
- *Match your leadership style with the competences of the staff*
(Blanchard et al, 1987).
- *Learning may be painful* or result in painful awareness of
inadequacies of expertise, resources or manpower; therefore, a
supportive climate is essential (Reddy, 1987; Tschudin, 1987).

TEACHING ISN'T TELLING

In this part of the chapter, we will look at ways, other than the didactic approach, of teaching in the clinical area. No doubt you are familiar with many of the ideas for increasing knowledge, developing skills and nurturing professional attitudes, but by considering them in a little more detail, they will be in the forefront of your mind and be ready for use in a variety of clinical situations.

Supervision

Pembrey (1980) identified failure to manage the ward, including management of the staff, as being the cause of trained nurses working together on the one hand, students working together on the other, and sister nursing patients on her own. In Pembrey's study, valuable opportunities for trained nurses to supervise students were lost. Students working together received no feedback on their performance and were possibly perpetuating mistakes or bad habits. Jacka and Lewin (1987) found that trained nurses estimated that they performed practical procedures with student nurses for 16.3% of the student nurses' time in the wards, while student nurses estimated that they were supervised by trained staff for 12.1% of their time. However, sisters estimated that the proportion of the student nurses' time on duty that was supervised by trained staff was 46%, while they thought that they spent 32% of their time in supervision!

White (1986) writes that people's results vary in direct proportion to management's interest in them. This aspect has already been touched upon in Chapter 1 in relation to organisational influences, and in Chapter 2 in connection with research findings. Fiedler et al (1976) propose that there are different leadership styles for different jobs, and this has been supported in more recent literature such as that of Blanchard et al (1987) and McCloskey and Molen (1987).

Therefore, what practical tips are available to assist a nurse with increasing the effectiveness of supervision as an aid to learning?

- *Manage by knowing your staff as individuals.*
- *Allocate trained nurses to work with untrained*, and more experienced with less experienced.
- *Set clear aims and give adequate instructions*, so that all know what is expected of them.

• *Treat your staff as members of a team*, not just as workers. White (1986) writes that treating somebody as a second-class person will never get first-class results.

• *Expect all members to do their best* and support them so that they can do it; praise them when they have done the task, even if all the work is not done. People can only do their best, and it is your job as manager and supervisor to facilitate their efforts.

• Having supervised a nurse carrying out a procedure or providing care for a shift, *give feedback*, otherwise no learning will take place (see the Law of Effect and the Law of Exercise, Appendix I).

• *Be constructive, not destructive.* Always avoid platitudes and insincerity, and if someone has carried out a procedure incorrectly, explain what and why it was wrong, and how it should be done. It is of no help to point out a nurse's shortcomings without indicating how she can improve her performance.

• However bad a performance, having pointed out the weaknesses and possible remedies, *try to finish on a positive note*, since there must be something good you can say. Destroying a person's confidence will be of no help to anyone concerned, and is more likely to inhibit learning than to enhance it. Read the section on reinforcement in Appendix I. White (1986) provides check-lists, exercises and points to consider for improving supervisory skills.

Some hospitals operate a mentor system for student nurses – that is, in each clinical placement a student is allocated to one qualified nurse, who has been given some additional training in the skills of mentoring and who will assess, together with the student nurse, her learning needs and abilities. As far as possible, the trained nurse and the student will together plan the experience to be gained, bearing in mind the need to provide care for the patients. The trained nurse will then assess the student's progress while, in addition, acting as mentor, supervisor and counsellor.

Role Reversal

One way in which to help a staff nurse prepare for a sister's post is to enable her to act as sister for a day while the sister is also on duty and can take the staff nurse's role. This needs a little planning, because patients and staff will automatically approach the sister if she is there, so forewarning of all concerned is advisable. In this way, the staff nurse can develop her skills without being thrown in at the deep end (Farnish, 1985).

Role Modelling

The work of Marson (1982) and Ogier and Barnett (1986) quoted in Chapter 2 has highlighted the importance of the role model in nurse learning. Remember that, even when no formal 'teaching' is taking place, staff are being influenced by the care given, how the ward is managed and how they are supervised. This awesome responsibility is carried by the qualified nurse for the future generation of nurses; therefore, be clear on your own standards – set them high, but realistically so. Role modelling plays a crucial part in the learning and development of attitudes, as may be seen from the following account.

In order to give them an inkling of what nursing is about, a group of new entrants to nursing had spent the afternoon in different clinical areas observing the various activities. They were asked what had impressed them most. Repeatedly, they gave examples of trained nurses showing caring understanding of the needs of a patient or relative, and the nurses' ability to communicate with the ill or the distressed, to allay fears, and not to be disgusted by unpleasant sights or behaviours. Attitudes take time to describe or explain, but are quickly demonstrated by every action and word. (See Appendix I for a summary of Bandura's, 1977, social learning theory.)

Small Group Discussion

Small group discussions form a useful way of fostering learning in the clinical area, but do need some thought and preparation. Gathering together a group of nurses at random for a discussion is bound to fail, and is more than likely to end up as 'a moan session'. Have a clear aim or purpose for forming the group – for example, a brainstorming session to get bright ideas for altering the layout of the patients' day room, or to pool knowledge on a specific topic, or to plan a research submission. Make clear what is expected of the group and by when it is required.

The value of a small group (six to eight people) is that everyone can contribute, ask questions and be participative. A little planning is necessary to consider the content and format of the group and its work, also its venue. The venue can make or mar a discussion; therefore, it is important to try to find a room where there will be no interruptions. Constant callers and bells ringing can disrupt the thread of the discussion and inhibit nurses from airing anxieties or possibly controversial views. Seating arrangements are important. If meaningful participation is to take place, it is necessary to arrange the accommodation so that each person can see the others face to face. As with all teaching and learning, attention to Maslow's hierarchy of needs will pay dividends (Maslow, 1970). Nurses who have missed lunch (Astbury, 1989), who are too hot or too cold, or just too tired, cannot be expected to function at higher levels of the hierarchy. Having some tea, coffee or fruit juice available may be helpful, but some health authorities have strict policies about where staff may eat and drink, so this should be checked beforehand.

Small groups are ideal for considering emotional, ethical or sensitive issues, about which nurses may hold various opinions. Pure factual knowledge can be imparted in a formal lecture or be gained by reading a book; however, some facts need to be presented as part of a discussion, to which they are more likely to form the background. For example, in a discussion on abortion, information on what the term means, what the Abortion Act (1967) says, why abortions are carried out and how many are carried out in the health authority may be provided. Like all teaching and learning activities, the aim of the discussion should be made clear to all participants at the start of the discussion or beforehand, so that the nurses can make an informed decision about joining the group. Clarifying the aim of the discussion also acts as a stimulus, preparing members so that they can begin to focus upon the topic and be ready to share and respond. Participation by all members of the group does not necessarily happen of its own accord: one member may dominate, or another may take the opportunity as a time to sit down, without any intention of exerting any energy in contributing. It takes skill to keep the group on the topic and to ensure a balance so that all members can speak. Do not *force* the quiet member to contribute. People have different learning styles and the quieter member may be thinking through the issues. Try an open encouraging question, such as, 'What do you think about . . .?' It may be far more difficult to control the garrulous member!

Patient-centred group discussion occurs when a willing patient explains why he is being cared for at home or in hospital, and puts forward his view of his illness or disability to a group of nurses, who can increase their understanding by discussing it with him.

Small group tutorials occur where one person, teacher, member of staff or learner, presents information on a chosen topic or on a patient care plan to other members of the staff. The opportunity to share, question and discuss in a small group in a non-threatening environment enhances learning, both for the presenter and the participants. By holding these sessions in the clinical area, discussion/learning is often felt to be more relevant and meaningful.

A good time for holding such small group discussions is when two shifts of nurses overlap. The changeover report between morning and afternoon shift is often extended to include more detailed accounts of patient care, many sisters using this time as a 'teaching report'. However, a word of caution: any overlap of staff will not necessarily be of use for learning or staff development unless there is a definite plan. Brykczynska (1988) carried out a study of the educational use of overlap time. She asked 217 nurses in one health authority how they actually spent the overlap time, and what would be the best use of it. There was disagreement between sisters and student nurses on how the time was actually spent, and they did not share the same ideal goals. Student nurses said that they mainly spent the overlap time relieving for meals and doing odd jobs, while sisters maintained that the students were giving direct patient care, or were involved in discussing care and learning with ward staff. In relation to ideal goals, sisters would like nurses to carry on giving direct patient care, but the student nurses saw the overlap time as an ideal time to attend ward tutorials given by ward staff. Brykczynska shows that the overlap time is not utilised for educational activities, and there is no reason to think that other health authorities differ from hers in this respect.

Teaching a Practical Skill

So far, we have looked at teaching that involves knowledge and attitudes, but nursing is very much a practical activity, especially so in general nursing. Before leaving the subject of teaching in the clinical area, it is important to consider briefly how a skill is taught or learnt there. Quinn (1988) provides a description of the theoretical background to learning a skill. Here it is proposed to provide a list of suggestions for teaching a skill in the context of patient care. The example chosen is teaching a student nurse to remove clips from a wound after surgery. The list applies equally well to teaching a nurse to apply an occlusive dressing to a leg ulcer, or to a staff nurse learning how to connect a patient to a cardiac monitor.

1. Specify what is to be learnt and how it fits into the overall care of the patient. In this example, it is the removal of clips from the neck wound of Mrs Gallez, who had a partial thyroidectomy three days previously. Explain that Mrs Gallez was suffering from thyrotoxicosis, which made her extra anxious, and that the operation was carried out to reduce the amount of gland and, therefore, the amount of thyroxin being produced. Explain also that surgeons often use clips to close neck wounds, as these have been found to result in less residual scarring.
2. Establish what the nurse already knows; for example, is she familiar with basic dressing technique?
3. Demonstrate preparation of the necessary equipment.
4. Gain the co-operation of the patient, and her permission for a student to observe the procedure.
5. Demonstrate the whole procedure, introducing yourself and the student nurse to the patient, explaining what happens when the clips are removed, leaving Mrs Gallez comfortable and afterwards clearing away.
6. Give the student the chance to ask questions.
7. Away from the patient, demonstrate the parts that go to make up the whole procedure: the preparation of the patient, both mentally and physically, preparation of equipment, the use of the clip removers, how they are held and, by opening out a clip, how they work. Indicate the 'teeth' on the clip which hold the skin edges together, so that the student can understand why the clip has to be opened out and eased from side to side, rather than lifted straight up.
8. At each point encourage the student to ask questions.
9. Allow the student to handle any unfamiliar equipment.
10. Arrange for the student to practise away from the patient, by removing clips from a sandbag that is covered in old sheeting.
11. Provide feedback on practice and allow further questions.
12. Demonstrate the whole procedure again.
13. Obtain permission from another patient for the student to remove her clips under your supervision and guidance. Supervise the student who is carrying out the procedure.
14. Give feedback on performance.
15. Encourage any further questions.

Depending on the complexity of the task and the ability of the student, be prepared to repeat any or all of the above until the student is competent. However, if the student is struggling to understand and master the skill, and you have checked that there is no obvious cause for the difficulty (for instance, she may not understand your diction), it may be better to leave the session for a day or two and then return to it afresh. The student may be suffering from information overload, trying to take in too much at once, or may be unwell, tired or anxious. This is where your skills as a sensitive, caring person are deployed in judging when to repeat and press on, and when to rest and provide time for consolidation.

Writing about influences on staff development, Heath (1987) says that more learning opportunities could be made available in the areas where people work. This chapter has tried to bring to the front of your mind, and increase your awareness of situations that may provide learning opportunities, and to consider some aspects of teaching in the clinical area. Telling does not mean teaching, and teaching is not necessarily telling. Learning involves all the senses, as demonstrated in learning a skill: receiving instruction (hearing), handling the equipment (touch), and seeing the layout and watching the procedure (sight), etc. Feelings will also influence learning, as already discussed.

In the next chapter we shall look at some ideas for teaching in the clinical area.

References

Alexander M F (1982) Integrating theory and practice in nursing – 1. *Nursing Times*, Occasional Papers, **78**(17): 65–66.

Argyris C and Schön D A (1976) *Theory in Practice: Increasing Professional Effectiveness*. San Francisco: Jossey-Bass.

Astbury C (1989) *Stress in Theatre Nursing*. London: Scutari Press.

Bandura A (1977) *Social Learning Theory*. New Jersey: Prentice-Hall.

Bendall E (1972) *So You Passed Nurse*. RCN Research Series. London: Royal College of Nursing.

Blanchard K, Zigarmi P and Zigarmi D (1987) *Leadership and the One Minute Manager*. Glasgow: Fontana/Collins.

Brykczynska M (1988) *An Evaluation of the Educational Use of Overlap Time*. Abstracts, Research Society Annual Conference April 1988. London: Royal College of Nursing.

Burnard P (1987) Teaching the teachers. *Nursing Times*, **83**(49): 63–65.

Cox C (1984) Editorial: Special issues, Developments in nursing education. *International Journal of Nursing Studies*, **21**(13): 151–152.

Deane D and Campbell J (1985) *Developing Professional Effectiveness in Nursing*. Reston, Virginia: Reston Publishing Co.

Douglass L M (1980) *The Effective Nurse*. St Louis: C V Mosby.

Farnish S (1985) How are sisters prepared? *Nursing Times*, Occasional Papers, **81**(4): 47–50.

Fiedler F E, Chemers M M and Maher L (1976) *Improving Leadership Effectiveness: The Leader Match Concept*. New York: Wiley.

Fretwell J E (1982) *Ward Teaching and Learning: Sister and the Learning Environment*. RCN Research Series. London: Royal College of Nursing.
Fretwell J E (1985) *Freedom to Change. The Creation of a Ward Learning Environment*. RCN Research Series. London: Royal College of Nursing.
Heath J (1987) Who and what influences staff development. *Senior Nurse*, **7**(6): 17–19.
Hunt J (1974) *The Teaching and Practice of Surgical Dressings in Three Hospitals*. London: Royal College of Nursing.
Jacka K and Lewin D (1987) *The Clinical Learning of Student Nurses*. NERU Report No. 6. Nursing Education Research Unit, King's College, University of London.
Jones D (1988) Looking beyond the boundaries. *Senior Nurse*, **8**(1): 26.
Knowles M (1984) *The Adult Learner: A Neglected Species*, 3rd edn. Houston: Gulf Publishing Company.
Lathlean J (ed) (1988) *Research in Action: Developing the Role of the Ward Sister*. London: King's Fund Centre.
Lelean S R (1973) *Ready for Report Nurse?* RCN Research Series. London: Royal College of Nursing.
Marson S N (1982) Ward sister – teacher or facilitator? An investigation into behavioural characteristics of effective ward teachers. *Journal of Advanced Nursing*, **7**: 347–357.
Maslow A H (1970) *Motivation and Personality*, 2nd edn. New York: Harper and Row.
McCloskey J C and Molen M T (1987) Leadership in Nursing. *Annual Review of Nursing Research*, **5**: 177–202.
Ogier M E (1982) *An Ideal Sister?* RCN Research Series. London: Royal College of Nursing.
Ogier M E (1986) An ideal sister – seven years on. *Nursing Times*, Occasional Papers, **82**(2): 54–57.
Ogier M E and Barnett D E (1986) Sister/staff nurse and the nurse learner. *Nurse Education Today*, **6**: 16–22.
Orton H D (1981) *Ward Learning Climate*. RCN Research Series. London: Royal College of Nursing.
Pembrey S (1980) *The Ward Sister – Key to Nursing*. RCN Research Series. London: Royal College of Nursing.
Porritt L (1984) *Communication: Choices for Nurses*. Edinburgh: Churchill Livingstone.
Quinn F M (1988) *The Principles and Practice of Nurse Education*. London: Croom Helm.
Reddy M (1987) *The Managers Guide to Counselling at Work*. London: British Psychological Society/Methuen. ·
Rogers J and Lawrence J (1987) *Continuing Professional Education for Qualified Nurses, Midwives and Health Visitors*. Peterborough: Ashdale Press.
Schmieding N J (1987) Face-to-face contacts: exploring their meaning. *Nursing Management*, **18**(11): 82–86.
Tschudin V (1987) *Counselling Skills for Nurses*, 2nd edn., ch. 11. London: Baillière Tindall.
Tough A (1979) *The Adult's Learning Projects*. Toronto: Ontario Institute for Studies in Education.
White J (1986) *Successful Supervision*, 2nd edn. London: McGraw-Hill.
Wilkinson J M (1985) *Moral Distress in Nursing Practice: Experience and Effect*. Unpublished MSc thesis, Kansas City, Missouri.

4
Some Teaching Ideas for the Clinical Area

Some specific ideas for learning in the work-place are the subject of this chapter. These are not original ideas: some stem from traditional theories of learning and teaching, some from management and leadership literature, and some are ideas that ward sisters have devised to enable their staff to keep up to date and growing in expertise. It might be wise, first of all, to realise that staff are individuals, since they have different complexions and different likes and dislikes, and therefore learn best in different ways. Learning styles have been identified by various researchers in education, and, in more recent years, nurse educationalists have begun to consider learning styles; notwithstanding that this chapter is about learning in the clinical area rather than in the classroom, it is still worth considering the different ways in which people learn.

Exercise

How do you learn? Do you like reading quietly and working it all out, or do you prefer to try out your ideas, share them with others, and so on? Describe your preferred ways of learning and ask some of your colleagues to do the same. Ask a few non-nurses how they learn best, because nurses may have been moulded or conditioned to respond in one particular way. Now identify and list the different ways that have been described.

Main (1985) described four learning styles, outlining how an individual with a preference for a particular style will learn best. Briefly they are:

1. *The Activist*
    – learns *best* from new experiences, change, excitement and involvement with other people;
    – learns *least* from lectures, reading and following precise instructions.
2. *The Reflector*
    – learns *best* when able to stand back from events and observe, consider and produce results in her own time, without tight deadlines;
    – learns *least* from being forced into the position of leader, from having to follow cut and dried instructions or from any situation which cannot be planned.
3. *The Theorist*
    – learns *best* from intellectual stretching, the use of models and concepts, and from analysing situations;
    – learns *least* when the topic is without purpose or too shallow.
4. *The Pragmatist*
    – learns *best* when she can link theory with practice and have immediate opportunity to implement what has been taught;
    – learns *least* when theory is removed from reality, when there are no clear guidelines and no chance to practise.

There are other ways of classifying learning styles, but the styles listed above are examples which highlight the fact that individuals learn best in different ways; therefore, when considering learning in the clinical area, it is necessary to look at a variety of approaches.

Garity (1985) reviewed the literature relating to learning style and various behaviours, such as leadership and learning. She concludes:

> 'In a shrinking economy nation wide, but particularly in health care, the future will belong to those who can successfully anticipate problems, build information networks and create bridges of shared resources with other disciplines. Continuing study of nurses' learning styles, with emphasis on demonstrated strengths and limitations, could provide valuable information to nursing leaders and educators that may assist greatly in addressing today's more pressing task in health care: reordering priorities and reallocating resources.'

Although Garity wrote this in the USA, it might well be applied to the UK, where there is an urgent need to ensure that nursing efforts are focused on where they are needed.

Ramprogus (1988), in the UK, investigated student nurses' learning styles and their problem-solving abilities. He found that student nurses generally do not show any preference for a particular learning style. This may be due to the type of nurse training they have been following, so that any variations in learning styles have been trained out of them. However, he did find that by giving the student nurses training in learning how to learn, there was a significant improvement in their learning performance and problem-solving abilities.

These findings are similar to those of Sookhoo (1988), who, as there is now a move towards a student-centred curriculum, decided to research the learning styles of student nurses by using the work of Kolb and McIntyre (1979). He found that different learning styles did not result in different learning processes. Again, does this result reflect the rigidity of the nursing world, where conformity is crucial and militates against independent thinking and problem-solving skills?

As mentioned in the previous chapter when discussing group work, student nurses are individuals and will learn in different ways, so that part of the initial assessment of student nurses should include an identification of their learning style. The learning experience can then be planned to maximise appropriate opportunities, thereby enhancing performance.

However ingenious and useful an idea may be, it will not bring forth the desired results of improved performance and learning if the climate of the work-place is not propitious to learning; therefore, a review of what has been written in earlier chapters may be helpful in relating the more general concept of learning climate to specific ideas.

Exercise

As a refresher or reminder, write short notes on what you remember to be the key issues in creating an environment in which it is safe to learn.

The following are some of the qualities which help to create a learning climate in the work-place:

- Know your staff.
- Appraise their abilities.
- Encourage them to 'own' the need to learn.

- Support them, so that they can identify their learning needs and set their own goals to meet those needs.
- Be 'open' to your staff, share with them your experience and expertise without dominating.
- Have a flexible leadership style to match the differing members of your staff: control, motivate, support, and delegate as appropriate.
- Encourage them to support you and each other so that you work together as a team.

Wright and Taylor (1984), writing about improving leadership performance, identified eight possible reasons for performance problems. It is worth considering the first seven of these as practical ideas for improving performance and learning in the clinical area. The final factor, *working conditions*, has already been covered in previous chapters. (Wright and Taylor's headings are in bold type, practical ideas in italic.)

1. Goal clarity: awareness of job requirements. As has already been discussed, some nurses may need help to see the need for updating, learning new material or revising long-held beliefs and values. *Give guidance on the standards they are expected to achieve, work to be completed, desired attitudes, philosophy of care for your unit, etc.* Nurses will then know what is expected of them and what they have to do to:

- meet the standards:
- develop the skills;
- exhibit appropriate attitudes.

Knowles (1984) identified the importance to the adult learner of setting clear goals. Burnard (1987) builds on Knowles' work, relating it to nurses and describing the value of establishing learning contracts, because individualising learning facilitates self-directed learning. If there is no current ward or unit philosophy, and if the staff have not agreed their learning activities:

- *write a philosophy of care for the ward/unit;*
- *negotiate learning contracts with the staff.*

Writing a philosophy of care can be a learning experience in several ways, because it helps to clarify ideas, values and beliefs. It may also help to formulate a theory of practice as discussed earlier (Argyris and Schön, 1976), and, as Deane and Campbell (1985) advocate, a theory of practice will help professional effectiveness and competence to evolve.

Ask your nurses to write down what they think is the philosophy of the unit. Looking at their responses may be an eye-opener, in that the staff's objectives may vary widely. There may be differences of opinion, expression or emphasis, and they may have ideas for practice that are more appropriate or up to date than those already in existence. Talk through the different ideas with the nursing staff, discuss what the ideas mean and how they could affect the work of the ward. The discussion will provide an opportunity for all the nursing team to learn and share. A common philosophy may have to be negotiated, which may then form the baseline from which all the nursing staff can work. With an agreed common philosophy, it should be much easier to establish each person's role in fulfilling that philosophy and in setting achievable, realistic goals.

It is now possible to move on to setting learning contracts with the members of the nursing team who will, if they know where they are trying to go, stand a chance of moving forward and getting there!

A learning contract is based on the learning needs of the individual; that is, the learning that has to take place if the gap between his or her present levels of achievement and skill and what these may or should be is to be filled. Negotiate the contract with the individual, help her to develop it; the importance of ownership has already been discussed. In a simple learning contract there are four steps.

The first step is to *identify the need*.

The second step is to *write down learning objectives*, that is, to state in meaningful terms what is to be learnt. It may be helpful to all concerned to state a period of time within which the learning is to take place. Specifying an agreed time limit has several virtues; it:

- prevents procrastination;
- provides a focal point for reviewing progress;
- may provide a priority of learning first those things which are the most urgent.

For example, a staff nurse newly appointed to the hospital may negotiate her first learning objective to be as follows: that by the end of her first week she should know and be able to tell a new student where the emergency equipment is stored and the correct procedure for an emergency, such as a cardiac arrest or a fire within the unit. At the end of a month she would be fully conversant with the care of a patient with, say, glaucoma (she would identify a patient whose needs were new to her nursing experience), and be able to assess, plan and carry out the care he required.

The third step is to *specify the learning methods* which are to be used. For example, the staff nurse learning the emergency procedures in a new hospital might:

- read the hospital manual;
- arrange for a member of staff to show her where the relevant equipment is stored and, if necessary, how to use it;
- visit co-ordinating areas such as main reception, hospital telephone exchange, and so on, in order to see how an emergency call is acted upon by other departments;
- attend in-service training related to emergency procedures.

Regarding her second objective of learning about the care of a patient wth glaucoma she might:

- arrange first of all to work with an experienced nurse, to observe the planning and giving of the necessary care;
- arrange to plan and give the care under the supervision of the experienced nurse;
- obtain relevant textbooks and articles from the library or ward;
- work through a self-teaching pack related to the objective;
- visit the post-basic education department to find out what relevant study days, seminars or other courses she can attend.

The fourth step is to *check that the learning contract has been fulfilled*. In the first example, the sister in charge may observe the new staff nurse while she explains and shows a new student nurse the correct procedures and the storage of the emergency equipment. In the second example, the staff nurse will have to demonstrate her proficiency in assessing, planning and caring for a patient who is suffering from glaucoma. In addition, and by prior agreement, the staff nurse's understanding of the needs of the patient, the possible treatments, complications, and so on, might be assessed by an experienced nurse, who would observe her giving a small tutorial to a group of student nurses on the care of patients with glaucoma.

The learning contract is specific to that nurse, and should be written down, agreed and signed by both the nurse and ward sister or nurse teacher, depending on whom her contract has been negotiated with. The effort necessary to develop a worthwhile learning contract will not only motivate the nurse by demonstrating a concern for her development, but will also provide a means of establishing clear goals.

2. Ability: has the person the ability to do the job? Issues related to formal appraisal and informal assessment of the nursing staff have already been highlighted. Once it has been decided that someone has a deficit, it is necessary to identify, together with the individual, how best that deficit can be reduced. *Ensure that the person has had the necessary training to undertake the work or particular tasks.* This is reinforced by the UKCC Code of Conduct (1984) which clearly states:

> '4. Acknowledge any limitations of competence and refuse in such cases to accept delegated functions without first having received instruction in regard to those functions and having been assessed competent.'

The American Nurses Association Code for Nurses with Interpretive Statements (1985) provides similar guidance:

> '6.2 . . . If the nurse concludes that he or she lacks competence or is inadequately prepared to carry out a specific function, the nurse has the responsibility to refuse that work and to seek alternative sources of care based on concern for the client's welfare . . .'

Be prepared, therefore, for the nurse who will require more training and, *where necessary, ensure that this nurse has supervised practice* until she is deemed to be proficient.

3. Task difficulty: the task is too demanding. Many people can remember instances when it seemed that they were trying to do or learn the impossible, but then someone came to the rescue and suggested ways of breaking the task down and gradually mastering it one step at a time. Where tasks or learning are difficult, *help the learner to divide the task into manageable chunks.* Allocating six patients to a second-year student nurse may provide her with an apparently insurmountable amount of care to be planned and given, but with guidance she can identify priorities, such as who is the most ill and needs immediate attention, who has to attend another department and therefore needs to be adequately prepared, who can safely be left to attend to his own needs, etc. Then work can be planned and carried out.

4. Intrinsic motivation: is the task rewarding in itself? Or, in the context under consideration, is the learning to be undertaken rewarding? Some nurses do enjoy learning for its own sake, but it may be that the majority undertake learning for the extrinsic benefits of better patient care which it will bring. Learning can bring self-esteem and personal growth in the enjoyment of having achieved a particular skill or reached a certain level of understanding. The reward of being able to achieve is the triumph, rather than performing the skill or demonstrating the knowledge. *Try to create a joy in learning accomplished and skills mastered,* a joy in the achievement and sense of development that learning can bring. Value the nurse who strives to improve her knowledge and skills while she is developing caring attitudes. As mentioned earlier, Rogers and Lawrence (1987) found that nurses who showed the most loyalty towards patient care were those most likely to continue learning. All nurses are individuals and, as individuals, have different abilities. One nurse may have to work really hard to achieve less than another; the important factor is that every nurse should do her best constantly to improve her efficiency and effectiveness.

   5. **Extrinsic motivation: good work rewarded by others.** One powerful motivator that stimulates nurses to learn is the need for good patient care. Gaining knowledge, mastering skills and developing attitudes conducive to a high standard of nursing motivate many nurses to expend a considerable amount of their own time and energy in further development and education. At present in the UK there is no financial reward for increasing expertise, although reward may come through increased job prospects. It may not be possible to alter the present state of affairs and reward learning by increased salary or job status, but you should *recognise and acknowledge the effort that members of your team are putting into developing their expertise.* Remember that, as mentioned earlier, personal recognition does much to improve morale and individual self-esteem.

   6. **Feedback: does the person get feedback on performance?** This topic has already been mentioned. *Do the members of your team know how they are performing?* This ties in closely with the first point raised by Wright and Taylor (1984), that of having clear goals. If the goals are clearly defined, it is then much easier to know whether or not a person has reached them, and to give specific feedback in progress towards those goals. Indeed, if the goals are clearly defined, people will probably know for themselves how they are progressing. This is one of the conditions necessary for adult learning depicted by Knowles (1984). It is very hard to be constructive when giving feedback to someone who is not performing as she should be if there are no clear, agreed goals to be reached.

   The importance of accurate, current feedback is highlighted in a letter written by Student Nurse Buxton to the *Nursing Times*

(Buxton, 1987). This letter also emphasises the importance of supervision and the feeling of being part of the team, aspects discussed in Chapter 3.

Being Honest on the Ward Report

'Excuse me, Sister, I shall be finishing on the ward on Saturday and I want to remind you about my ward report.'

'Goodness me, Nurse, can't you see how busy I am?' says Sister, bustling off to make sure the beds are made correctly.

One week later, in her own time and at the fourth attempt, Nurse Brown says, 'Good afternoon, Sister, I'm sorry to bother you but I still . . .'

'Yes, yes, your report Nurse – Nurse er . . .?'

'Yes, of course, Nurse Brown. Here we are now. We'll just fill in a little something by the initial interview and the mid term one. Don't go letting them at the school know, will you?'

'Nurse Brown is settling nicely and working reasonably well', she writes and says, 'Now then just a few boxes to tick. If you'd just like to sign the bottom.'

Nurse Brown looks longingly at the space marked 'learner's comments' and thinks, 'If I put what a poor learning experience I really think it was it'll look like sour grapes after such a mediocre report. Anyway I can feel her beady eyes daring me to write something critical.' So hurriedly she writes:

'An enjoyable experience. I shall be sorry to leave.'

'Thank you, Sister', says Nurse Brown, and races out of the office.

The solution? Some more boxes for the learner to answer the following:

I was introduced to the ward on my first day
I was made to feel part of the ward team
I was given supervision whenever necessary
I was able to meet my ward objectives
I was able to implement individualised patient care
I was encouraged to question practices I felt unsafe or not research-based
I was able to devote time to the psychological as well as physical needs of my patients.

Just the sight of the boxes might be enough to prompt sisters to review their attitude, ward practice and level of support for learners. If not, a few statistics compiled from such reports and forwarded as a matter of course to nursing officers might do the trick.

The learner had the right to her comments, too, and has a right to make them away from the intimidating gaze of the ward sister. Nurse Brown really can help improve the level of patient care in the wards, but she needs to be given the opportunities and the support mechanisms to do so.

(Reproduced by kind permission of the *Nursing Times*, where this letter first appeared on 18 November 1987)

Student Nurse Buxton is not alone – anecdotal reports from sisters and students reiterating the views and feelings expressed in this letter are frequently heard. What valuable learning opportunities are being lost! If the student was working only 'reasonably well', it is not surprising, since without an initial interview, was she unaware of what was expected of her, and without feedback during the allocation, how did she know that she needed to improve? What is more, as Student Nurse Buxton finishes her letter, what a pity for the patients not to receive care from a nurse performing at her best.

Sister said that she was too busy to do the student's report, a common cry heard from sisters around the UK: 'We have no time'. How long do a word of welcome and an introduction to the ward take? How long does it take to complete the interim report? Weigh up the time spent with the student against the time lost through her ineffective work, while she is trying to find things and to discover what is expected of her. What a pity it is to have a student in your area for 8 to 12 weeks who is functioning below her full potential! Surely a lot of time is lost during this period – no wonder sister didn't have time, for it was being frittered away.

7. **Resources: are there enough to do the job satisfactorily?** Resources are finite, and in the late 1980s definitely shrinking, so rather than raise the demand for greater resources, let us look at what resources are available and think of ways by which they can be maximised to aid learning in the clinical area.

Exercise

Make a list of all the resources of which you are aware that can be utilised to assist learning and professional growth in the clinical area in which you work.

At the top of the list should be personnel, i.e. you and the other nurses. The enormous influence that the role model has for good or bad has already been discussed in previous chapters. Reddy (1987) writes that people are the most important asset of any business, and that failure to value them and ensure their effectiveness makes the company less successful. The crucial effect that the leader of the nursing team has on creating a favourable environment for learning has also been considered.

If all the resources such as videotapes, books and tape-and-slide presentations are available, but the person in charge does not value learning, it is more than likely that the staff will not use these resources. Unless the work situation is managed with sensitivity, opportunities will be lost and staff will be stifled and their development cramped, with the leader or manager's own growth being curtailed.

Reddin (1987), who writes about developing an effective management style, says that low situational sensitivity is often due to low style awareness. In preceding chapters, it has been suggested that you question yourself and your values and beliefs, developing a theory of practice, so that you are in touch with yourself as a professional worker. The need to be approachable and to be open to others has been discussed; perhaps in this practical section it might be wise to question how you know if you are approachable, and how you can become more approachable and 'open'. Reddin provides a management-style diagnostic test at the beginning of his book. Alternatively, you may like to ask yourself how the nurses in your ward or department would complete the following statements about you. (If you are a staff nurse, substitute 'Staff Nurse' for 'Sister', or use your own name.)

Circle one of the five words presented to complete each statement:

1. *Sister makes sure that I know what to do*: always, often, sometimes, occasionally, never
2. *Sister makes sure that I know how to do what she asks*: always, often, sometimes, occasionally, never
3. *When I don't know something, Sister makes sure that she (or someone) tells me how to do it or find out about it*: always, often, sometimes, occasionally, never
4. *When I am worried or don't know something, I feel that I can go and ask Sister*: always, often, sometimes, occasionally, never
5. *I feel that I can talk to Sister*: always, often, sometimes, occasionally, never
6. *Sister is interested in me*: always, often, sometimes, occasionally, never
7. *Sister is helpful to me*: always, often, sometimes, occasionally, never

These questions are drawn from the Learners Perception of Ward Climate (LPWC) questionnaire developed by the writer in a study of the role of the ward sister, and now in use in the UK, Eire and Iceland. It was found that, on the whole, sisters did have realistic perceptions of themselves when their responses were compared with the responses of nurses on the wards.

You may wish also to ask the nurses who work with you to complete these statements, but before you do so, talk over the idea with a trusted colleague, because you may get responses which you do not like and you will need her support to talk through the findings and your feelings about them.

The best way to receive an honest response and realistic feedback is by ensuring that the nurses do not identify themselves by name on the questionnaire, and that they themselves place the completed questionnaire in a box or envelope.

If you are approachable, the majority of the nurses in the ward will circle 'always' or 'often' to each of the seven statements. For your interest, Table 4.1 shows the percentage of nurses who replied 'always' or 'often' for the ideal sister and 'occasionally' or 'never' for the non-ideal sister, during the period when the questionnaire was being developed. Similar findings have been obtained subsequently on numerous occasions, the most recent being in April 1987.

Table 4.1 Approachability of the ideal and non-ideal sister

Question:	1	2	3	4	5	6	7
Ideal (approachable) sister							
Always or often	95	85	95	82	77	70	82
Non-ideal (unapproachable) sister							
Occasionally or never	75	72	67	90	87	81	87

It can be seen from the table that over two-thirds of nurses responded 'always' or 'often' for sisters who were approachable, while for least-preferred sisters, over two-thirds of the nurses thought that they were definitely not approachable, because they only occasionally or never demonstrated the relevant behaviours.

In addition to providing some questions to ask yourself and, perhaps, your staff, the questions also highlight the behaviours that demonstrate your approachability. Your ability to communicate effectively is a crucial part of approachability. Marson (1984), in describing the good teacher in the clinical area, identifies three important components:

- the power of the role model;
- skill in forming and managing interpersonal relationships;
- the art of being a good communicator.

Some aspects of ward communication that have already been considered in earlier chapters are:

- ensuring clear and unambiguous nursing prescriptions and instructions (Lelean, 1973; Pembrey, 1980);
- fostering constructive participation in decision-making and problem-solving (Schmieding, 1987);
- discussing skills of communication such as active listening (Porritt, 1984; Reddy, 1987). (These texts provide down-to-earth, practical advice and help for the clinical nurse and/or manager.)

The importance of competent leadership has been discussed previously, and some aspects related to developing leadership skills in the clinical area have been brought together in a short article by Ogier (1984), which, in addition to many of the aspects already covered, highlights empathy and humanity. Carkhuff (1973) defines empathy as the ability to understand another person and to be sensitive to his or her needs. Porritt (1984) writes that someone who shows empathy is able to respond caringly to another person, accepting the other's feelings without judgment and without the need to solve her problems for her. Being empathetic means being involved in, but not swamped by, another's experience, as happens in sympathy. Empathy means involvement with the retention of personal boundaries. This results in effectiveness, for, despite hearing and understanding something of what the other person feels, the emotions are not overwhelming, so a helpful response can be made. By allowing someone to express her feelings and values, without evaluating them, that person can be helped to look at her own situation and develop possible solutions to her problems. As Schmieding (1987) advises, do not rush in and solve people's problems, but give them the space and support to find their own solutions, thereby aiding their personal growth and development. Caring understanding can facilitate learning. One indication of being empathetic is the willingness of staff to approach their ward sister.

It is not necessary to be the fount of all wisdom, but rather to be the creator of a learning climate in which others are able to contribute. Do not try to alter or improve all skills and behaviours at once, otherwise exhaustion is likely and nothing will be achieved. Take one aspect at a time – such as your decision-making skills, listening skills or leadership style – and work on it. A list of useful publications that may help you to consolidate your expertise will be found in the Further Reading section at the end of this book.

Nurses do not work alone, so how can other trained nurses act as a resource to aid learning? A new staff nurse from another hospital may be a resource, first, by bringing different ideas and perspectives to common issues, second, by bringing new information, and third, by looking at the clinical area with fresh eyes, often noticing aspects which have gone undetected or unquestioned. Student nurses can act as a powerful stimulus by asking, 'Why do you do that?', 'Why does that happen?'

By encouraging each nurse to take specific interest in a particular aspect of care, for example in care of the elderly, one nurse may develop a special concern for the care of patients suffering from Alzheimer's disease, whereas another may have a particular aptitude for helping those who suffer from dysphasia. By following the nurses' particular interests, by asking them to contribute to discussions and share information with other members of the staff, and by asking them to provide a teaching session for the student nurse, and so on, the nurses involved will have a sense of being needed, as they demonstrate a level of expertise and act in a consulting capacity to their colleagues, rather than seeing themselves just pairs of hands. They contribute to the body of knowledge on the ward and their self-esteem is increased, which in turn enhances the likelihood of their further development. Furthermore, ward morale rises, and satisfied nursing staff are more likely to remain in post, thereby not depleting scarce manpower resources.

Sadly, there is a shortage of manpower in the NHS, and it is likely to get worse; one health authority estimates that by 1996 there may be a 45% vacancy level (North East Thames Regional Health Authority, 1987). Thus it is important to utilise the available staff to the utmost and enable them to develop their full potential, not only for their own personal growth but also for the well-being of patients, clients and the organisation.

Other personnel are also involved in the clinical area – physiotherapists, occupational therapists, behavioural therapists, clinical psychologists, chaplains and others – and can share their expertise with the nurses and explain their contribution to patient care.

In addition to the most precious resource – people – other resources are available in the clinical area or may be borrowed, and can be used to assist with teaching and learning. These include some of the following items.

Tape/slide presentations are commercially available on a vast number of nursing, medical and related topics, and are often obtainable in or through the school or college of nursing. One value of such presentations is that the only equipment necessary is a cassette recorder and a slide viewer, which can be small and hand-held, or full size for classroom use. The majority of nurses are familiar with the working of cassette recorders and slide projectors from their own personal use of them, so they are not put off by technicalities. The hand-held viewers are small enough to be used in clinical areas, and, together with cassettes, they can be easily stopped and started if the nurse is called away. Thus, tape/slide sets represent a useful way of deepening or extending knowledge. Although the clinical area is likely to be busy, there may be periods during the day when there is a lull in the work, for example at visiting time or when shifts change over, when a tape/slide presentation can be used by one or all of the nurses. The majority of tape/slide presentations are not long: most last for less than 35 minutes, and it is quite possible to look and listen for shorter periods. Difficult or unusual material can be returned to time and time again, therefore being adjustable to nurses' different learning styles and abilities. As these materials can be used at any quiet moment in the 24 hours, they are, therefore, valuable for night nurses and part-time staff.

Videotape recordings of nursing and medical topics are also available, and while these are not so easy to employ in the clinical area, there are places and times when their use will be feasible.

Self-teaching packages are available from distance learning centres or from the Open University. Again, the education centre or school of nursing may have copies that can be borrowed. Teaching packages allow the individual to work at her own pace, and, for some nurses, present a less threatening medium than do seminars or study groups, where the nurse may fear that she may be put on the spot by being asked a difficult question.

Notice boards are possibly the most unused, disregarded form of communication: they are rarely read and little or no notice is taken of the information displayed thereon. However, some sisters have used notice boards to good effect in the clinical area, with good attention paid to them by the nursing staff.

One such sister calls her notice board a 'topic board', and, together with the nurses of that ward, she has drawn up a list of topics relevant to the ward and of interest to the staff. Every 2 weeks she puts the title of one of the topics on the board, and each member of the staff is expected to contribute a 'piece' related to that topic. Such a 'piece' might be a comment from a women's journal, a newspaper, a professional journal or a textbook; it can be drug information, information about medical equipment and/or supplies from manufactures' representatives, or a project that the nurse may have completed on a course. Note that this sister has involved the staff by identifying areas that are of interest to them, and then by encouraging each person to contribute, providing support and encouragement where necessary. The sister found that a period of 2 or 3 weeks for each topic allowed enough time for everyone to participate and read the others' contributions, so that even nurses with days off, those who were on night duty and part-time staff had the chance of updating, again without threat and at their own pace. At the end of the specified period, the material was taken down and stored for future reference in a file on the ward. The list of topics was made easily accessible to the staff, so that they could save material from newspapers or journals for use with future topics.

Another sister had a similar idea but organised it in a different way. Staff identified topics in which they were interested, and the sister allocated the board to each nurse in turn for 2 weeks. During that period, the nurse could display material that she had collected on her chosen area of interest. Again, it was available for all staff, including part-time and night staff, to read. It could have happened that the other nurses 'switched off' and showed no interest when it was not their turn, but the sister reported that since all nurses, part-time and night staff as well, were invited to participate, group pressure resulted in their showing interest in each presentation, since they knew that their turn would soon come. Likewise, a few nurses were reluctant to participate, but, again, when they realised that it was a fairly painless procedure (even if it required a certain amount of early planning to gather the information as it came along), they took their turn. Once more there appears to be an additional benefit in improved morale and a raising of awareness of professional issues and current clinical knowledge.

It is important to make sure that the notice boards are placed where patients do not have easy access, for, while patients are now being encouraged to become better informed about their conditions, there are more appropriate ways of informing them.

For example, should the newly diagnosed diabetic read a list of all the possible complications and see photographs of gangrenous limbs? It could be disastrous for his well-being and compliance with treatment.

Journal clubs. These may be arranged at ward level, between a group of wards or for the whole hospital or community, and they may be multidisciplinary or just about nursing. Small, work-related journal clubs can be very beneficial. Because time is limited, it is common to find them being held during the lunch-break, when members bring a packed lunch and then share pertinent points from their reading. There is now a multitude of nursing journals, and no one person can be expected to read or even scan them all. With each nurse buying a different journal or reading it in the library, and then meeting others to share a summary of any material relevant to the ward or current professional issues, there is a chance that every member will keep abreast of the welter of information being produced. There is an additional motivation which helps the nurse to keep up with her reading, for by being part of a group, she will let the rest of the group down if she does not read her allotted share. It is so easy to put off reading, especially after a busy day, and the magazines pile up until they become such a big heap that they are altogether too intimidating to start on, and it is easier to cancel the subscription!

Nurse's journal or diary. In some schools of nursing and as part of some post-basic nursing courses, nurses are encouraged to keep a journal or diary of events, feelings, problems and their solutions, and such like. Burnard (1988) describes how the use of a journal can form part of a nurse's assessment. However, the use of a journal in the clinical area can help the nurse to review her own progress and highlight areas of interest as well as any difficulties. While it is possible for the nurse to use the journal as a self-monitoring device, it may be of more use if several nurses in the same area each complete a journal and share their ideas and experiences.

The above suggestions gleaned from other nurses may have provided some ideas or support for the plans already formulated. Bearing in mind the constraints of time and lack of resources, the focus has been on the facilities and ideas that are likely to be available now but are often underused, possibly owing to the lack of an environment where learning is valued and seen as an essential ingredient for patient care of a high standard.

References

American Nurses Association (1985) *Code for Nurses with Interpretive Statements.* Kansas City, Missouri: American Nurses Association.

Argyris C and Schön D A (1976) *Theory in Practice: Increasing Professional Effectiveness.* San Francisco: Jossey-Bass.

Burnard P (1987) Teaching the teachers. *Nursing Times*, **83**(49): 63–65.

Burnard P (1988) The journal as an assessment and evaluation in nurse education. *Nurse Education Today*, **8**(2): 105–107.

Buxton V (1987) Being honest on the ward report. Letters, *Nursing Times*, **83**(46): 15.

Carkhuff R R (1973) *The Art of Helping.* Amherst, Massachusetts: Human Resource Development Press.

Deane D and Campbell J (1985) *Developing Professional Effectiveness in Nursing.* Reston, Virginia: Reston Publishing Co.

Garity J (1985) Learning styles: basis for creative teaching and learning. *Nurse Educator*, March/April: 12–16.

Knowles M (1984) *The Adult Learner: A Neglected Species*, 3rd edn. Houston: Gulf Publishing Co.

Kolb D A and McIntyre J M (1979) *Organisational Psychology: Readings in Human Behaviour in Organisations*, 4th edn. Englewood, New Jersey: Prentice Hall.

Lelean S R (1973) *Ready for Report Nurse?* RCN Research Series, London: Royal College of Nursing.

Main A (1985) *Educational Staff Development.* London: Croom Helm.

Marson S N (1984) Developing the 'teaching' role of the ward sister. *Nurse Education Today*, **4**(1): 13–15.

North East Thames Regional Health Authority (1987) *Strategy for the Education of Nurses, Midwives and Health Visitors.* London: North East Thames RHA.

Ogier M E (1984) Developing leadership. *Nurse Education Today*, **4**(1): 8–11.

Pembrey S (1980) *The Ward Sister – Key to Nursing.* RCN Research Series. London: Royal College of Nursing.

Porritt L (1984) *Communication: Choices for Nurses.* Edinburgh: Churchill Livingstone.

Ramprogus V K (1988) Learning how to learn nursing. *Nurse Education Today*, **8**(2): 59–67.

Reddin W J (1987) *How to Make your Management Style More Effective.* London: McGraw Hill.

Reddy M (1987) *The Manager's Guide to Counselling at Work.* London: British Psychological Society/Methuen.

Rogers J and Lawrence J (1987) *Continuing Professional Education for Qualified Nurses, Midwives and Health Visitors.* Peterborough: Ashdale Press.

Schmieding N J (1987) Face-to-face contacts: exploring their meaning. *Nursing Management*, **18**(11): 82–86.

Sookhoo D (1988) *Approaches to Studying Adopted by Student Nurses.* Abstract, Research Society Annual Conference. London: Royal College of Nursing.

United Kingdom Central Council for Nursing, Midwifery and Health Visiting. (1984) *Code of Conduct for the Nurse, Midwife and Health Visitor*, 2nd edn. London: UKCC.

Wright P L and Taylor D S (1984) *Improving Leadership Performance.* Hemel Hempstead: Prentice Hall.

5
Have Courage to Learn

God grant me the *serenity* to accept the things I cannot change,
the *courage* to change the things that I can and
the *wisdom* to know the difference. (Anon.)

Learning requires a change of behaviour for many qualified
nurses and this, in turn, may require courage. Brookfield (1986)
writes that, for change to take place, students must be adequately
motivated and aware of the inadequacy of their present
behaviour. To admit one's shortcomings or weaknesses does
take courage, yet nurses have the best possible motivation in
their constant desire to provide a quality service to the ill, the
old and the vulnerable. The preceding chapters have considered
various ideas and activities for facilitating learning, based on
the assumption that the more quickly and efficiently learning
can take place the better, not only for the those learning, but
also for the well-being of patients and clients. Pembrey (1987)
holds the view that continuing education is essential for real
change in clinical practice, while King (1986) states that change
has become a way of life as we look toward the twenty-first
century. Change has increased anxiety, but education is seen
as a way to cope with it. Change is inevitable, but change and
education do go hand in hand. There are three options:

- Change can be initiated, which is based on professional
  knowledge and clinical expertise.
- Change can be accepted by adapting and assimilating the
  changes that others initiate.
- Change can be resisted at all cost, thus using up precious
  resources of time and energy in trying to maintain the status
  quo.

Some changes initiated by nurses in the light of research
findings have been mentioned already, such as those of Pembrey
(1980), who, having completed her research into the management
style of the ward sister, returned to the clinical area to implement
her findings and developed a successful training ward for ward

sisters. Fretwell (1985), who had identified wards that were not conducive to learning in her first study (1982), implemented a change programme using action research, to enable the staff to create an environment within which it was safe to learn. Alexander (1982) tried to reduce the gap between theory and practice by means of an educational experiment. Bryant (1985), who identified that the ward sisters in her study were unaware of the nurse training curriculum, established a training programme for the sisters to help them to become more conversant with the curriculum and learners' needs (the original studies have been described in Chapter 2).

It may be tempting to think, 'It's all right for those people – they are probably senior nurses or nurse researchers; I'm only an ordinary, busy clinical nurse'. However, Lathlean (1988) recounts how ward sisters developed ideas and implemented changes in their work areas following presentations of research findings. Take heart! Have courage to learn through change, and, through learning, initiate and support change.

What attributes or abilities do you need to be able to implement change? Ogier and Barnett (1985) replicated Ogier's earlier study of ward sister leadership styles and their effect on learners in the clinical area, and extended it to examine how the sisters were coping with change as they introduced the nursing process. It was found that sisters who had been successful in implementing the nursing process had high 'consideration' and high 'structure' scores, as measured by Fleishman's Leadership Opinion Questionnaire (LOQ; Fleishman, 1969) (see Table 5.1). High consideration scores indicate that the leader creates a climate of good rapport and two-way communication. High structure scores characterise an individual who plays an active part in directing group activities through planning, communicating information, scheduling, criticising and trying out new ideas, in fact, all the characteristics that are essential if change is to be introduced.

The sisters who were least successful in introducing the nursing process in their areas had either low consideration and structure scores or just low scores on structure. Having regard to the definition of structure, this might be an expected finding, so in order to assist the sisters to introduce change, it was necessary to help them to become more active in planning, criticising and giving information. However, the study did highlight a potential problem, one sister being required to demonstrate two leadership styles. In Chapter 2, the sisters whom learners rated most highly were described as having high

Table 5.1 LOQ scores for sisters ranked on success of implementing nursing care plans for individualised patient care; presented with type of ward and ranking of learner preference for sister as measured by LPWC, ranked for each type of ward

	Most successful									Least successful				
LOQ														
Consideration	67	60	60	70	55	48	53	55	60	51	53	56	58	61
Structure	53	54	45	49	48	46	32	33	40	42	46	44	35	45
Type of ward	M	S	M	M	M	Sp	M	M	M	M	S	M	M	S
Learner ranking	5	5	9	1	2	1	3	7	6	4	8	8	10	7

M=medical ward, S=surgical ward, Sp=paediatric or geriatric

(Reproduced by kind permission of *Nursing Times*. This table first appeared in *Nursing Mirror* on 17 July 1985)

consideration but a level of structure that was appropriate to the nature of the work. In unfamiliar, stressful areas of nursing, learners tolerated higher levels of structure than in areas where they were more familiar with and confident about the work required of them. If the sister is required to increase her structure levels to be successful in introducing change, what happens to the learning environment in that area? If, as was indicated at the beginning of this chapter, there is a need for change and that change is inevitable, how is the learning climate to be protected? Most of the learners in the study had forged alternative support systems for themselves, mainly with the staff nurses, but rather than let learners seek help and support in a haphazard fashion when a change is to be introduced, be alert to:

- the changes needed in leadership style in order to facilitate successful change;
- the needs of the students, and the need to compensate for the changed leadership style and to ensure that the learning climate is maintained.

Remember that once the change has been implemented a revision of leadership style may be necessary. The 'ideal sister' identified by Ogier and Barnett (1985) was the sister who was able to alter her style to match the introduction of change by becoming more active in planning and communicating information, but once the change had been implemented was able to revert to a structure score which was appropriate for that clinical area.

Change is a time for teamwork and support from senior nurses, as was clearly described by Fretwell (1985). Race (1987), in a preliminary report of a study into the effectiveness of continuing education for ward sisters, writes that participants benefit most when the ward sister and her manager have common objectives for the course, and that the project work for the course should arise from the sister's real work and should have realistic aims. Results are also better when the manager is willing to support the ward sister in her effort to implement changes. Race also emphasises some of the issues already discussed, i.e. realistic aims, clear objectives, learning related to working and adequate support from the management and the organisation.

Breu and Dracup (1976) were anxious to introduce change in nursing activities in a critical care unit. The spouses of patients admitted to coronary care had expressed dissatisfaction with certain aspects of care, especially where their needs had not been met in relation to their seriously ill spouse, highlighting aspects such as the need to be with the dying person, and the need to be helpful and of assistance to him. Breu and Dracup also recognised that it would be necessary to formulate a plan for change. The work of Lewin (1958) had demonstrated that organisational behaviour is not static – rather, it is a dynamic balance of psychosocial forces working in opposite directions. Lewin called the forces that tend to increase the possibility of change 'driving forces', while the forces that depress change or movement were called 'resisting forces'. Therefore, for change to take place, there are three possible strategies:

● increase the driving forces by adding new forces or strengthening existing ones;
● reduce or remove resisting forces;
● translate one or more of the resisting forces into driving forces.

With knowledge of the work of Lewin, and building on the eight principles of Klein (1968), Breu and Dracup introduced a new nursing care plan to meet the needs of the spouses of critically ill patients. Since their work provides a clear example of how clinical nurses can apply theory and research findings to change strategies for the benefit of patients, it is worth considering it in some detail. As you read on, why not make a note of the points and use them to assess the likelihood of introducing change in your work area?

1. *There is an almost universal tendency to seek to maintain the status quo on the part of those whose needs are being met by the present situation.* For example, Breu and Dracup established that there was instability in the unit that they studied, because the head nurse had left and had not yet been replaced, hence the need to maintain the status quo and not increase the instability by introducing change.

2. *Resistance to change increases in proportion to the degree to which the change is perceived as a threat.* The threat identified by Breu and Dracup was the anxiety that staff felt in helping others with death and grief and in dealing with their own feelings toward death. The staff's unfamiliarity with research was also perceived to be threatening. Adequate support and time to talk through issues reduced some of the threat.

3. *Resistance to change increases in direct response to pressure to change.* As Breu and Dracup were, respectively, clinical specialist and clinical teacher to the unit, it could have been perceived by the staff that the change was being forced upon them by people in authority; therefore, time was spent in explaining the voluntary nature of the participation with the changed care plans for spouses.

4. *Resistance to change decreases when it is perceived as being reinforced by trusted others, such as high-prestige figures, those whose judgment is respected and people of like mind.* Again, open communications with all concerned helped, as did the fact that both Breu and Dracup were known and respected in the unit.

5. *Resistance to change decreases when those involved are able to foresee how they might establish a new equilibrium as good as or better than the old.* This relates to, 'Why change?' Because staff in the unit had identified the needs of the families of the dying, the change was seen as trying to improve the situation.

6. *Commitment to change increases when those involved have the opportunity to participate in the decision to make and implement the change.* In the study being discussed, participation was high from the beginning. As highlighted in Principle 5, the staff had identified the initial need and were involved in offering ideas for change.

7. *Resistance to change based on fear of the new circumstances is decreased when those involved have the opportunity to experience the new under conditions of minimal threat.* By using an initial experimental phase of pilot study, staff could try the proposed

change, assess the benefits and make alterations before the change was adopted permanently.

8. *Temporary alterations in most situations can be brought about by the use of direct pressure, but these changes are accompanied by heightened tension and will yield a highly unstable situation.* Hence, careful planning, with adequate time for consultation with all concerned, is essential.

The eight principles which have been outlined here (with examples from the work of Breu and Dracup) can be applied to any work situation for any change, however small or large. Time spent considering these aspects will be recouped in the easier implementation of the change. More recently, Robinson (1987) looked at the uptake of research findings by ward sisters. Her conclusions support many of the aspects discussed above. Robinson writes that new knowledge is often threatening to practitioners, since it may threaten practices that have been carried out, satisfactorily from the practitioner's point of view, for many years. Robinson continues:

> 'To suggest that there may be another way of doing something is to imply that researchers, who after all are not concerned with immediate day-to-day problems of running a hospital or ward, are saying that what has been done in the past is somehow inappropriate or even downright harmful and therefore practices must change.'

In the light of such perceived threats, Robinson concludes that it is not surprising that practitioners reject research findings and claim that as it is they who do the work, only they can be expected to know what is best.

Describing a study of the preparation of nurse tutors, which included an understanding of the use of the nursing process, Hollingworth (1985) writes that the introduction of the nursing process has been the most fundamental change in nursing in recent years. It was in 1977 that the General Nursing Council stated, in a policy document, that the nursing process provided a unifying thread for the study of patient care and a useful framework for nursing care. Five years later, Hollingworth reports that half the nursing schools in her study were not teaching the nursing process or planning to do so. The overwhelming factor that was stopping the adoption of the nursing process was the lack of understanding of the concept of individualised care and its implications for practice and education. Hollingworth continues that this highlights a major weakness in the nurses' claim to professional status, namely the failure to keep their knowledge and skills up to date. She recommends that there is an urgent need to establish a system of continuing education in nursing, to help nurses prepare for the change and to develop an awareness of the need for a personal commitment to keep up to date with professional knowledge.

In a more recent study, Hale (1987) comments that while it is obvious and desirable that care should be organised to meet the needs of individuals, it is not clear how this can be achieved when there are few nurses and many patients, especially when care is given in an institution. The aim of her study was to introduce, and then examine the effects of, a change in the method of organising the delivery of care in one ward of a maternity hospital. Prior to the study, the work in this ward was mainly task-centred, and the change to be introduced was a method of giving care which would be patient-centred. Hale found that the patients had a high level of satisfaction with their care prior to the changes, so that it was hard to measure an increase in satisfaction following the change!

Abdellah (1987), when writing about setting standards in clinical practice, says that although change is not easy, nurses must recognise and take advantage of the opportunities it offers. Nurses need to recognise trends in nursing; then they will be proactive in developing creative responses. One of the impending changes is the restructuring of nurse education, which is being formulated in the UK (UKCC, 1987). Jones (1988) says that all nurses share the responsibility of innovations in nurse education, and that the essence of nursing is learning on-the-job while working with skilled, competent practitioners. The practitioners will need to know about student-centred learning, problem-solving and new learning methods; some of these aspects have already been mentioned. Bratton (1987) has compared the problem-solving process with the nursing process and with 'instructional development process', and has highlighted that all three follow the same seven steps:

- Collect information.
- Diagnose.
- Develop a plan or solution.
- Implement the plan or solution.
- Evaluate the effects of the solution or intervention.
- Decide whether the action was adequate.
- Recycle through the process.

Before groaning or feeling that here is yet another idea/model or process to be mastered, stop and look at the principles involved. Instead of thinking that you have to start afresh with a new idea, remember that similar skills and abilities can be applied to similar tasks or activities (Cognitive Theories, Appendix I). Bratton proposed that the ability required to care for a patient can be applied to helping another nurse to learn by:

- finding out what the nurse's learning needs are, that is, by gathering appropriate information about what she already knows and where gaps exist in her knowledge;.
- planning the teaching/learning session, whether demonstrating a particular procedure or giving supervised patient care;
- carrying out the planned session;
- evaluating – checking whether the nurse has learnt, and whether it was what was intended;
- deciding if her learning and the teaching are adequate; have her learning needs been met, and has the plan been fulfilled?

If necessary, the cycle can be repeated.

By using familiar principles from the problem-solving process or the nursing process, learning in the work-place can be enhanced and the teacher will gain confidence. The student nurse not only learns but also feels that her needs are recognised, thus furthering self-esteem and growth.

Introducing change uses a similar process, but change does not occur without resistance, as highlighted by Breu and Dracup (1976), and discussed by Allan (1987) and Docking (1987) when considering resistance to innovation in the curriculum. Wright (1985) describes the successful introduction of change, with the implementation of the nursing process in the care of the elderly. This was achieved by the use of one person who acted as the change agent. Pembrey (1987) warns that even after change has taken place, it is fragile until it has been accepted and become the norm.

How can the busy clinical nurse have the courage to learn, initiate change where necessary and cope with the resistance to innovation that seems to be inevitable? Having considered some of the reasons for resistance to change and some of the stages of the change process, a few practical tips or activities will now be discussed.

Lewin's (1958) classic theory of change provides a useful framework within which to consider how best to initiate change.

It identifies three stages in the change process:

- *unfreezing*, which happens when there is motivation to make a change, perhaps due to the acquisition of new knowledge;
- *moving*, which involves planning and initiating the change;
- *refreezing*, which occurs when the change is integrated into the system.

Nurses in one health authority introduced a professional model of nursing in which the individual nurse enters into a relationship with her own patient, is responsible for and accountable to that patient and can defend her decision and actions as being in the patient's best interests (Pembrey, 1987). This requires knowledgeable, rational skilled nursing. Pembrey outlines the stages followed in the process of introducing the innovations, which are:

- creating the climate;
- planning for the change;
- educating for the change;
- implementing the change;
- sustaining the change.

Each of these stages will be briefly considered.

In order to *create a climate for change*, there needs to be a focus person, preferably with a recognised role and status in the organisation. This person may be appointed specifically as a change agent, or may be the ward sister or staff nurse. The function of the focus person is to co-ordinate the various activities, to gather information and ideas and to communicate with, and elicit support from, other personnel. As discussed in earlier chapters when addresssing the issue of creating a learning climate, sensitivity to others, together with a sound knowledge base, is essential if a climate of change is to be accomplished. The very fact of seeking information and ideas from the staff helps them to begin thinking about a particular topic. Committed support from seniors is crucial in building a non-threatening environment in which innovation can take place, and where staff are prepared to take part in innovative process.

Planning for change involves gaining support and co-operation of colleagues, peers and subordinates as well as seniors, planning the stages of the change, arranging a pilot scheme, disseminating information and educating where necessary.

Educating for change is not only concerned with developing the skills of a change agent and the ability to communicate clearly and motivate others, but also includes the education related to the change itself, such as the philosophy of individualised care or, as in Pembrey's (1987) case, the professional nursing model.

Implementing the change. It is essential to have clear aims and guidelines, so that all those involved know what they are trying to achieve and what their part is in the whole.

Sustaining the change. Pembrey warns that even after a change has been accepted and is being widely used, it may still be sabotaged by lack of support from key people. Sustaining the change may be as hard as implementing it, requiring supportive networks to be developed.

Some reasons why people resist change have already been mentioned. A few of these are: it is easier to carry on with the familiar; change may be threatening in several ways – it may challenge long-held beliefs and values, or may show up areas of weakness such as lack of skill or knowledge; change threatens because it results in uncertainty and ambiguity, and there may be a fear of loss of control in unfamiliar territory.

All these points give rise to anxiety and stress, and that in itself is another barrier to change. However, before jumping to the conclusion that someone is resisting the innovation just because it is a change or because it challenges their abilities, stop and *listen* to what they have to say and to their ideas. The crucial nature of real listening was discussed in a previous chapter: listen to the *message*, not just the words. The person resisting you may have considered seriously and objectively all aspects of the change and made a rational, well-informed decision to oppose the change. Listening and paying attention to what she has to say may save a lot of time and effort. She may be right! The change may be inappropriate, or it may need to be modified in the light of her comments. It follows, therefore, that not all resistance to change is bad, for it can be helpful in assisting the clarification of ideas and in developing a case for change, ensuring that the change is appropriate for the situation. The silent resister is far more difficult to cope with; if she does not voice her dissent, it is impossible to furnish her with any more information or counteract her anxieties. Do not presume silence to be affirmation – check a silent member's views and opinions on the proposed change. By demonstrating a genuine interest in her contribution, time and effort may be saved by incorporating her ideas, where appropriate, into the innovation; it may even be possible to get her involved in the change. It takes a great deal of interpersonal skill to achieve the understanding and co-operation of the majority of people involved, but the effort will pay dividends in the future as the change process evolves.

Some practical tips and questions to ask when planning to introduce a change, however small or however radical, whether it is in the way the work is allocated or whether it is to make a change in nursing practice as a result of research findings, are as follows:

- *Be quite clear and specific about what it is that is to be changed.* Try writing down ideas and then sharing them with a trusted friend or colleague. The act of talking through ideas helps to clarify and refine them; after discussion it may be necessary to rewrite the original idea. Underline four to six key words as these will help to focus attention when searching for relevant information. (For a more detailed account see the sections on Finding Information and The Literature Search in Ogier, 1989.)
- *Make sure that the necessary knowledge, information and skills required by the change are available,* and, where possible, identify resources.
- *Collect and collate the relevant information into a short readable form,* so that it can be assimilated quickly by others who are also busy. If there is information that provides contrary evidence, that is, against the change, include it in the review. Presumably, despite the contrary information, the change is still to go ahead, in which case all involved need all the available information to enable them to make an informed decision. It is tempting, in order not to give ammunition to opponents of the change, to pretend that a counter-argument does not exist, but this is unwise. By presenting both sides of the argument, the case for change appears less biased. Failure to mention the contrary information will only enable opponents to raise that aspect, so it is better to acknowledge its existence and use it as part of a balanced argument.
- Having gathered together the information on what the change is about, there are questions to be answered before taking the ideas any further, as follows (some of these questions are those that will be asked when the proposed change is introduced, and it may be helpful to jot down the answers for use on that occasion):

  – *Why should there be change?*
  – *Is the proposed change for the better?*
  – *What is the aim of the change;* are there clear, realistic goals?

- *Who will be involved in the change?*
  - directly, such as patients and nurses;
  - indirectly, such as storekeepers, porters, disposal units, the nurse education centre, trade unions and others?
- *What are the costs and benefits, obvious and hidden?* For example:
  - the obvious cost are such things as new equipment, stationery or more staff, depending on the change you intend to make;
  - the hidden costs include lowering of standards while the new change is mastered, increased anxiety and sickness, more staff, time for training, and so on;
  - the obvious benefits include improved patient care and more efficient use of time and/or manpower;
  - the hidden benefits include such things as improved morale, the 'Hawthorne effect', improved team work, increased learning and staff development.

- At the end of the above exercise, a *succinct summary* of the proposed change, clear aims and realistic goals, with the costs and benefits weighed up, should be available. The proposed change can be introduced to seniors and staff with a view to obtaining their co-operation in creating the climate for change.
- *Identify people who will be part of the support and planning group.*

These suggestions are just the beginning of the process of introducing change. A sound knowledge of the material related to the change is needed, as well as the skills of a communicator and of a negotiator – besides those of being a supreme diplomat!

This chapter is entitled 'Have Courage to Learn' and much of the emphasis in it has been on change. Change is necessary for a person to learn and grow. Growth leads to increased knowledge and skills, professional attitudes and self-awareness, which in turn lead to the ability to identify areas that are in need of change. So, for a healthy nursing profession, which is essential for high standards of care, it is crucial to foster an environment where learning is a valued, integral part of work, because as Blanchard et al (1987) write:

'Everyone is a potential high performer; some people just need a little help along the way'.

It is hoped that this book will be a little help along the way. In the final chapter we shall look at a few issues related to measuring high performance, and finish with some self-evaluation and goal-setting.

References

Abdellah F (1987) Setting standards for clinical practice. *Nursing Standard,* Special Supplement, **2**(10): 4–5.
Alexander M F (1982) Integrating theory and practice in nursing – 1 and 2. *Nursing Times,* Occasional Papers, **78**(17 and 18): 65–68, 69–71.
Allan P (1987) The evolving curriculum in nursing education. In: *The Curriculum in Nursing Education,* Allan P and Jolley M (eds). London: Croom Helm.
Blanchard K, Zigarmi P and Zigarmi D (1987) *Leadership and the One Minute Manager.* Glasgow: Fontana/Collins.
Bratton B D (1987) Systematic planning for teaching and learning. In: *The Teaching Process, Theory and Practice in Nursing,* van Hoozer H L, Bratton B D, Ostmoe P M, Weinholtz D, Craft M J, Albanese M A and Gjerde C T. Norwalk, Connecticut: Appleton-Century-Crofts.
Breu C and Dracup K (1976) Implementing nursing research in a critical care setting. *Journal of Nursing Administration,* December: 14–17.
Brookfield S D (1986) *Understanding and Facilitating Adult Learning.* Milton Keynes: Open University Press.
Bryant R J (1985) *The Role and Preparation of the Ward Sister Involved in Nurse Training.* MSc dissertation, Department of Educational Studies, University of Surrey.
Docking S (1987) Curriculum innovation. In: *The Curriculum in Nursing Education,* Allan P and Jolley M (eds) London: Croom Helm.
Fleishman E A (1969) *Manual for Leadership Opinion Questionnaire.* Chicago: Science Research Associates Inc.
Fretwell J E (1982) *Ward Teaching and Learning: Sister and the Learning Environment.* RCN Research Series. London: Royal College of Nursing.
Fretwell J E (1985) *Freedom to Change. The Creation of a Ward Learning Environment.* RCN Research Series. London: Royal College of Nursing.
Hale C A (1987) *Innovation in Nursing Care. A Study of a Change to Patient Centred Care.* RCN Research Series. London: Royal College of Nursing.
Hollingworth S (1985) *Preparation for Change. Preparing Nurse Tutors in Initial Training for a Change to Nursing Process.* RCN Research Series. London: Royal College of Nursing.
Jones D (1988) Looking beyond the boundaries. *Senior Nurse,* **8**(1): 26.
King I M (1986) *Curriculum and Instruction in Nursing. Concepts and Process.* Norwalk, Connecticut: Appleton-Century-Crofts.
Klein D C (1968) *Community Dynamics and Mental Health.* New York: John Wiley.
Lathlean J (ed) (1988) *Research in Action. Developing the Role of the Ward Sister.* London: King's Fund Centre.
Lewin K (1958) The group decision and social change. In: *Readings in Social Psychology,* Maccoby E (ed.) London: Holt, Rinehart and Winston.
Ogier M E (1989) *Reading Research.* London: Scutari Press.
Ogier M E and Barnett D E (1985) Unhappy learners ahead? *Nursing Mirror,* **161**(3): 18–20.
Pembrey S (1980) *The Ward Sister – Key to Nursing.* RCN Research Series. London: Royal College of Nursing.

Pembrey S (1987) Achieving excellence through innovation. *Nursing Standard,* Special Supplement, **2**(10): 8–9.
Race A (1987) Effectiveness of continuing education. *Nursing Times,* **83**(48): 55.
Robinson J (1987) The relevance of research to the ward sister. *Journal of Advanced Nursing,* **12**: 421–429.
United Kingdom Central Council for Nursing, Midwifery and Health Visiting (1987) *Project 2000, The Final Proposals.* Project Paper 9. London: UKCC.
Wright S G (1985) Change in nursing: the application of change theory to practice. *Nursing Practice,* **2**: 85–91.

6
Where to Now?

This final chapter will consider a few aspects related to attaining professional excellence, providing high quality of care given by up-to-date, competent nurses.

Clay (1987), writing about the way forward for nurses, says:

> 'Excellence in preparation, by education, has to be the foundation for excellence in practice.'

He also says that nurses do know the way forward: it is about the right to nurse patients, the right to practise high standards of care and the right to a proper education. Jones (1988) believes that nurses have moved forward by a quantum leap:

> 'But we have argued for many years that nursing is more than simply a series of tasks carried out by reasonably intelligent individuals. It is therefore important that any new approach which we adopt should centre on the concept of caring for the total person, rather than simply treating the sick. I believe that we are moving along the right lines and have already taken a quantum leap in this direction.'

While Clay and Jones are fairly sure that nurses know where they are going and have made a start along the right path, it is likely that British nurses are no different from their North American colleagues. Cooper (1982) reviewed continuing education in North America and its implication for practice, and concludes that while there has been remarkable progress in continuing education during the last decade, the concept of lifelong learning for professional practice is not universally accepted by nurses. In a study of nurse education in the European Community, Quinn (1982) reports that the rate of development is uneven but that there are initiatives for continuing education. She concludes that there are opportunities, problems and frustrations, but whether or not the opportunities are seized and the problems and frustrations overcome depends on the nursing profession. The individual clinical nurse is not alone in striving to improve care – nurses in other units, hospitals, communities and countries are also working to improve the quality of the service provided for patients, despite shrinking resources and ever-growing demand. The problems appear to be universal, so how can learning be shared by nurses in order to help one another?

Some current nursing issues, such as individualised patient care through the nursing process, the valuing of the individual's rights and treating both patients and staff as 'whole' people with their own preferences, needs and abilities, have been raised in the preceding chapters. Success as a practising nurse, who is also a manager, an educator and an organiser, will depend on the skills of identifying individuals' needs and abilities and of creating an environment in which needs can be expressed and abilities nurtured. While it is essential to maintain care, nurses have constantly to strive to provide quality of care. As Swaffield (1987) writes:

> 'Quality is not just a fashionable buzzword, it is a concern which goes to the heart of nursing.'

Quality cannot be separated from individualised care that is planned, given and eveluted by competent, effective, accountable nurses. How is quality measured? How do nurses know whether the care they prescribe, supervise and give attains a quality that might be described as acceptable, good or even poor? When buying a new electrical appliance the purchaser is advised to look for the British Standards mark, and in other countries a similar mark indicates that the appliance has been tested and has met certain safety standards. Likewise, when booking into a hotel or guest-house it is usual to look at the establishment's rating – the number of stars or crowns – which measures the quality of service and furnishing that may be expected. What are the nursing standards against which to measure the service being provided? It is possible that one of the reasons why nursing is poorly valued and underrated is the lack of a clear definition of what nursing is and how it differs from what a caring layman might do. What criteria are used to assess nursing and its standards?

In 1981, the Regional Office for Europe of the World Health Organisation decided to launch a new programme called 'Model Health Care Programmes and Quality Assurance', the emphasis of which was on two issues:

- the most appropriate combination of services in the care of a patient with a given problem;
- the quality of health services.

Vuori (1982) writes that the best way to clarify what is meant by quality of health services is to divide the concept into four components:

- effectiveness;
- efficiency;
- adequacy;
- scientific/technical quality.

The importance of the nurse being both efficient and effective has already been discussed, and is one of the crucial aims of promoting nurse learning in the clinical area. Vuori defines adequacy by posing the question, 'Does it meet the patients' needs?' 'Scientific/technical quality' refers to the level of application to care of currently available medical knowledge and technology.

One way of approaching the complex task of assessing quality (Donabedian, 1980) is by considering:

- the structure, that is, the input and organisation;
- the process, that is, the content and configuration;
- the outcome, that is, the procedural end point or the impact.

This framework proved useful when helping community midwives to review the service that they provided. By preparing a grid of nursing process × quality assurance (Table 6.1), the midwives had a format within which to appraise the care that the mother received, using the same format to highlight their own role in each part, while identifying their strengths and weaknesses. The process was greatly facilitated by the availability of *Maternity Care in Action*, nos. 1 (1982), 2 (1984) and 3 (1985); these are guidelines from the DHSS which provide criteria for desired standards.

For clarity, only one or two items have been included in each 'square'; however, each square of the grid can be further elaborated and used to aid discussion among the midwives that is in itself stimulating and growth-promoting. For example, consider process/assessment: what choice of care is available to the pregnant woman – (a) consultant care and hospital delivery, (b) GP care and delivery in a domicillary unit and (c) home delivery. Does she know about these services, has she any choice and has she the necessary information to make a choice?

This system has the advantage of building on what the midwives already know of the concepts of the nursing process, acknowledges their expertise and provides guidelines for working step-by-step through a vast amount of information. (The

Table 6.1   Care appraisal – nursing process × quality assurance.

Quality assurance	Nursing process			
	Assessment	Planning	Implemen-tation	Evaluation
Structure (input)	Mother's age, health, risk factors, etc.	Programme of care, attendance at clinic, GP, etc.	Medical and obstetric checks.	Were risk factors detected?
Process	Types of care available	Adequate information, suitable care for mother	Attendance at classes, etc.	Were visits helpful?
			Informed consent	Were wishes respected?
	Delivery	Delivery plan	Transfer to hospital, etc.	Delivery safely completed?
Outcomes: immediate	Lochia Breasts Fundus Baby Apgar score, etc.	Postnatal checks	Check mother and baby	Uncomplicated puerperium? Baby developing?
final	Family unit	Health education	Alert HV	Is family unit functioning?

importance of 'achievable steps' has already been discussed in Chapter 3.) While the exercise was aimed at improving the quality of maternity care, considerable learning and growth were experienced by the participating midwives, since they were able to review their ability to provide the service that they identified as being needed. This was good for everyone concerned, even if the exercise was a painful one at times when long-held ideas were challenged; however, supportive teamwork ensured development rather than retardation.

Another way of considering quality by involving the people providing the service, namely quality circles, is described by Robson (1984), who writes that quality circles are an approach which allows employees to become more involved, by solving their own job-related problems in an organised way. A circle is composed of people involved in the work; for example, a quality circle for a ward for the care of the elderly might be composed of a staff nurse, an enrolled nurse, the occupational therapist and the social worker, and be facilitated by the unit manager or senior nurse. For the circle to work, Robson stipulates eight points:

1. Participants must really be volunteers, not people 'volunteered' by management or their peers. The volunteer, her manager and her supervisor all need to agree that she should take part.
2. The problem to be looked at must be the participants' own and not someone else's. For example, a problem owned can be: 'I have difficulty in planning my time in order to give each patient my attention at some point in the day'. Someone else's problem might be: 'Management does not increase my staff, so how can I be expected to see every patient each day', or 'Sister never does a complete round of all the patients, so those who are left out feel that they are unimportant'.
3. Problems have to be solved in an organised way, so this may require prior training.
4. Participants should meet for an hour once a week during working hours.
5. The facilitator of the circle should be in line management because he or she will have to:
6. take results to management.
7. Management may or may not act.
8. The circle should evaluate any action taken.

Several health authorities in the UK already use quality circles in various areas of clinical nursing.

One difficulty when considering quality and its assessment is that there are no clear criteria with which to contrast present work and to help to promote higher standards, other than those for midwives that have just been mentioned. McCall (1988), when discussing the evaluation of quality, points out that there is a tendency among nurses to use the terms 'quality' and 'standards' as if they are the same thing. She writes that standards are part of a package that leads to quality.

The Royal College of Nursing has been active since 1967 in trying to identify and measure the components of a quality nursing service. In that year, Baroness McFarlane of Llandaff led a team of researchers to study various aspects of nursing care. Several of their studies have already been mentioned in this book, for example, *Nil by Mouth* (Hamilton-Smith, 1972) and *The Teaching and Practice of Surgical Dressings in Three Hospitals* (Hunt, 1974), together with more recent monographs (see Chapter 2). In 1978, the RCN established a committee to look at standards of nursing care, which has produced the discussion document, *Towards Standards* (Royal College of Nursing, 1981). This document frequently stresses the need for nurses to have continuing education, in order that they may equip themselves to make the necessary changes to improve and maintain standards. The need for support by management is also emphasised. In 1985, the RCN established its Standards of Care Project, which, in addition to providing leadership and assistance on particular aspects of quality assurance to nurses throughout the UK, is developing specific projects yet to be reported on. However, the annual *Nursing Quality Assurance Directory* (Royal College of Nursing, 1987) lists the various initiatives being undertaken throughout the country to measure quality, to identify standards of care and to set criteria by which to measure care. Also available from the same source is a useful bibliography concerning quality of care.

In looking at the quality of care and students' educational experience in hospital wards, Smith and Redfern (1988) conclude that:

> . . .the relationship between quality of nursing and ward learning is articulated through the sister's emotional style of management.'

They found that patients judged the quality of nursing by the emotional style in which it was given, irrespective of the nature of their illness and the technical care that they required. Student nurses associated a good learning environment with wards that had a high patient turnover and patients with a variety of diagnoses requiring acute, technical nursing and specialist medical intervention. Smith and Redfern also reported that when the Quality Patient Care Scale (Qualpac) and participant observation were used, the quality of nursing 'was extremely difficult to measure objectively'.

So what can nurses giving care do, especially in a situation of widespread cutbacks and manpower shortages? They can work to improve their own knowledge, skills and abilities, so that they are better equipped to face the difficulties. Just as important as constantly striving to keep up to date, they can create an environment where staff can learn and gain confidence through a sound knowledge base with relevant expertise and professional attitudes, and will come to see continuing learning as an integral part of a quality service. In this way, the individual nurse will not be alone, but there will be a nucleus of keen, caring nurses.

It is to be hoped that this and the preceding chapters will have provided some practical ideas on how the work-place can be made conducive to learning without taking up scarce resources of time and manpower. As Easterby-Smith (1986) indicates, people who are developing are more likely to create opportunities in which to use their potential, because of their greater confidence and interest in learning.

The remaining pages include some questions and ideas to help you to clarify where you are now, where you are trying to go, how you will get there and how you will know when you have arrived. As individuals all have different needs, the headings encompass a variety of needs, allowing plenty of scope to personalise responses. After all, the exercises are intended for use as a guide and reminder of what you are hoping to accomplish, and their honest completion will prevent you from deluding yourself. Complete the inventory now and, in six months' time, look back at what you have written. It is easy, when you are busy, to feel that nothing has been achieved. The record can act as a base from which to identify what has been achieved, and as motivation to try afresh in areas where more can be achieved.

Having read this book, it should be possible to formulate answers to the following exercises without too much difficulty; the relevant sources or sections of the test are indicated. N.B. As these are self-assessment exercises, 'I' refers to *you*, the reader. Tick a column or delete inappropriate words as necessary.

Where are you now?

Current Personal Inventory

Today's date (as a record of when the exercise was started):
Present post:

As manager: (Chapter 2, The Sister as Manager)
I know my strengths to be:

I know my weaknesses to be:

continued next page

— continued —

My priorities are (Pembrey, 1980):

The following stop(s) me from working as I think I should in order to give the patients the best possible care:

I have taken the following action/no action in order to reduce or eliminate the above:

If you are a ward nurse: I do a round of all the patients for whom I am responsible each time I am on duty: always, usually, sometimes, occasionally, never
or
If you are a community nurse or work in a department, how do you identify priorities and assess needs?

(Tick the appropriate column)

	Always	Usually	Sometimes	Occasionally	Never
I give clear, specific, verbal nursing prescription to the staff for whom I am responsible					
The nursing orders I write are the same as the verbal nursing prescriptions (Lelean, 1973)					
I check that the staff know how to do what I ask (Ogier, 1982)					
I am aware of the needs and abilities of my juniors					

— continued next page —

continued

	Always	Usually	Sometimes	Occasionally	Never
I match the needs and abilities of my juniors and my peers with the needs of the patients					
I use research evidence in the management of patient care (Royal Marsden Hospital, 1984)					
I use research findings to support my negotiation and discussion					
I manage my time rather than managing by crisis, rushing from one task to the next (Adair, 1987)					
I *listen* to the staff in my area (Porritt, 1984; Reddy, 1987)					

Other comments about my management abilities:

As leader: (Chapter 2, The Sister as Leader)

My leadership style is usually (describe):

(Ogier, 1982; Blanchard et al, 1987; Reddin, 1987)

continued next page

continued

	Always	Usually	Sometimes	Occasionally	Never
The staff find me approachable (Ogier, 1982; Chapter 4)					
My leadership style suits junior staff					
My leadership style is appropriate for experienced staff					
I adapt my style to suit the situation (Ogier and Barnett, 1985; Chapter 3)					
I delegate effectively					

Other comments about my leadership:

As educator: (Chapter 2; Orton, 1981; Fretwell, 1982, 1985; Marson, 1982; Ogier, 1982, 1983, 1986)

Qualified nurses feel part of the nursing team					
Nurse learners feel part of the team while they work in my area					

There is a programme of continuing eduction in my area: Yes/No

All the nursing staff contributed to the development of the education programme: Yes/No

continued next page

continued

	Always	Usually	Sometimes	Occasionally	Never
I ensure that all staff have the chance to contribute to the education programme					
I ensure that all staff have a chance of attending continuing education that takes place in my area					
Educational activities outside my area are drawn to the attention of my staff					
I encourage and support my staff to attend educational activities beyond the area					
I encourage my staff to identify their own learning needs and then to seek suitable educational activity					
There is a close liaison between the basic nurse training school and my unit					
There is a close liaison between continuing education and/or training department and my unit					

continued next page

continued

In my unit there are (tick those that you have):

- Information packs/folders
- Up-to-date textbooks
- Topic board
- Discussion programme
- Journal club
- Audiovisual aids:

  - tape/slide
  - video
  - specify others:

	Always	Usually	Sometimes	Occasionally	Never
Each member of staff is involved in setting his or her own clear objectives with specific goals					
I meet individual subordinates to provide them with feedback and a chance to air their views (circle answer): at least every six months, once a year, less than yearly, never					
I use research-based evidence in the teaching that I undertake					

As role model, the attitudes which I wish to model are (Marson, 1982):

continued next page

106 Working and Learning

106   Working and Learning

---

106 Working and Learning

106 Working and Learning

106 Working and Learning

106 Working and Learning

106 Working and Learning

106 Working and Learning

106 Working and Learning

106 Working and Learning

106 Working and Learning

106 Working and Learning

106 Working and Learning

106 Working and Learning

106 Working and Learning

How are you going to get there?

Does your immediate manager know of your ideas and plans? This is strongly advisable as you will need to negotiate such matters as study leave. If you have a formal appraisal system it may include much of the ground covered by the exercises that you have just completed.

Have you made contact with your local continuing education department or training centre to find out what is available for you locally?

By reading a nursing journal relevant to your work, you will hear about courses, study days, seminars and new textbooks.

Look out for scholarships or funds for which you can apply, to help you to attend conferences or courses.

Do you belong to a professional organisation or union? These are another source of information, courses and funding.

What are the professional library facilities in your vicinity? Do you know what range of material is available in them? Most libraries have access to an enormous range of books through inter-library loan, so if you cannot see what you want, do not presume that it is unavailable. If it is your first time in the library, ask one of the staff to show you how to find the information you need.

As a clinical nurse, it is all too easy to concentrate on the care of the patients, to your own detriment, and in the long run this will affect them because you will gradually become more out of date.

Slack (1986) believes that the good potential ward sister should make her needs plain and seek jobs where top management is supportive, while Wainwright et al wrote in 1986 that many ward sisters are frustrated at having to ask middle managers about changes that they wish to make in their wards, decisions that *they* feel should rightly be *theirs* to make. In turn, middle managers are often hampered by their seniors, who try to retain control over them. Some of the factors that may influence a competent nurse who is looking for a new post might include:

- a continuing education programme with specified study leave entitlement;
- an open, responsive management that is willing to respond to enquiries about management structure and style.

How will you know that you have reached your goal?
In some ways there is no end to professional development and personal growth, because there are always aspects that can be developed and built on. However, it is necessary to evaluate progress. The exercises you have completed can form part of the evaluation, and, as already mentioned, the personal inventory can be completed again at six-monthly intervals, thus providing a self-assessment which indicates those aspects of your skills and abilities that have improved and those that still need to be worked on. For, as Easterby-Smith (1986) writes, there are three general purposes to evaluation: proving, improving and learning. Completion of the inventory now and after a further six months as a part of self-assessment aims to meet the purpose of improving and learning: improving, in the sense that efforts can be made to ensure that your future performance is better, and learning, in that by becoming more self-aware, your energies can be focused towards specific areas of need. The whole purpose of this book is to help qualified nurses to develop, that is, to have a greater ability to learn from the experiences available, which is where this book began. The need to learn *how* to learn is a sound foundation for professional competence. Indeed, Ramprogus (1988) has developed a manual to help nurses learn how to learn.

It is hoped that this book has made a small contribution to the effort of developing and maintaining professional competence. Mager (1968) was writing for teachers when he stated:

'One objective toward which to strive is that of having the student leave your influence with as favourable an attitude towards your subject as possible. In this way you will help him maximise the possibility that he will remember what he has been taught and willingly learn more about what he has been taught',

but it may be that his words apply equally to this book and the reader's efforts in the clinical area.

References

Adair J (1987) *How to Manage Your Time*. Guildford: Talbot Adair/McGraw-Hill.
Blanchard K, Zigarmi P and Zigarmi D (1987) *Leadership and the One Minute Manager*. Glasgow: Fontana/Collins.

Clay T (1987) The way forward. *Nursing Standard*, Special Supplement, **2**(10): 15.

Cooper S S (1982) Continuing education in nursing: implications for clinical practice. In: *Recent Advances in Nursing, 4: Nursing Education*, Henderson M S (ed.) Edinburgh: Churchill Livingstone.

Donabedian A (1980) *The Definition of Quality and Approaches to its Assessment*. Ann Arbor, Michigan: Health Administration Press.

Easterby-Smith M (1986) *Evaluation of Management Education, Training and Development*. Aldershot: Gower.

Fretwell J E (1982) *Ward Teaching and Learning: Sister and the Learning Environment*. RCN Research Series. London: Royal College of Nursing.

Fretwell J E (1985) *Freedom to Change. The Creation of a Ward Learning Environment*. RCN Research Series. London: Royal College of Nursing.

Hamilton-Smith S (1972) *Nil by Mouth*. RCN Research Series. London: Royal College of Nursing.

Hunt J (1974) *The Teaching and Practice of Surgical Dressings in Three Hospitals*. London: Royal College of Nursing.

Jones D (1988) Looking beyond the boundaries. *Senior Nurse*, **8**(1): 26.

Lelean S R (1973) *Ready for Report Nurse?* RCN Research Series. London: Royal College of Nursing.

Mager R F (1968) *Developing Attitudes Towards Learning*. Belmont, California: Fearon Publishers.

Marson S N (1982) Ward sister – teacher or facilitator? An investigation into behavioural characteristics of effective ward teachers. *Journal of Advanced Nursing*, **7**: 347–357.

Maternity Care in Action, 1 (1982), 2 (1984), 3 (1985). London: DHSS.

McCall J (1988) Evaluating quality. *Senior Nurse*, **8**(5): 8–9.

Ogier M E (1982) *An Ideal Sister?* RCN Research Series. London. Royal College of Nursing.

Ogier M E (1983) The ward sister as a teacher resource person. In: *Research into Nurse Education*, Davis B D (ed.). London: Croom Helm.

Ogier M E (1986) An 'ideal' sister – seven years on. *Nursing Times*, Occasional Papers, **82**(2): 54–57.

Ogier M E and Barnett D E (1985) Unhappy learners ahead? *Nursing Mirror*, **161**(3): 18–20.

Orton H D (1981) *Ward Learning Climate*. RCN Research Series. London. Royal College of Nursing.

Pembrey S (1980) *The Ward Sister – Key to Nursing*. RCN Research Series. London. Royal College of Nursing.

Porritt L (1984) *Communication Choices for Nurses*. Melbourne: Churchill Livingstone.

Quinn S (1982) Nurse education in the countries of the European community. In: *Recent Advances in Nursing, 4: Nursing Education*, Henderson M S (ed.) Edinburgh: Churchill Livingstone.

Ramprogus V K (1988) Learning how to learn nursing. *Nurse Education Today*, **8**(2): 59–67.

Reddin W J (1987) *How to Make your Management Style More Effective*. London: McGraw-Hill.

Reddy M (1987) *The Manager's Guide to Counselling at Work*. London: British Psychological Society/Methuen.

Robson M (1984) *Quality Circles in Action*. Aldershot: Gower.

Royal College of Nursing (1981) *Towards Standards*. London: Royal College of Nursing.

Royal College of Nursing, (1987) *Nursing Quality Assurance Directory*. London: Royal College of Nursing.

Royal Marsden Hospital (1984) *Manual of Clinical Nursing Policies and Procedures*. London: Harper and Row.

Slack P (1986) What future for the ward sister? *Nursing Times*, **82**(46): 28–30.

Swaffield L (1987) Quality assurance: every nurse's job. *Nursing Standard*, Special supplement, **2**(10) 2–3.

Vuori H V (1982) *Quality Assurance of Health Services. Concepts and Methodology*. Copenhagen: World Health Organisation.

Wainwright P, Brimelow A and Campen Y (1986) More than just Managing. *Nursing Times*, **82**(46): 30–32.

Further Reading

These are in addition to the texts referenced at the end of each chapter.

Nursing Education

Alexander M F (1983) *Learning to Nurse: Integrating Theory and Practice.* Edinburgh: Churchill Livingstone.
Royal College of Nursing (1982) *Research Mindedness and Nurse Education.* London: Royal College of Nursing.
Runciman P J (1983) *Ward Sister at Work.* Edinburgh: Churchill Livingstone.

Nursing Practice

Benner P (1984) *From Novice to Expert.* California: Addison-Wesley.
Burnard P and Chapman C M (1988) *Professional and Ethical Issues in Nursing.* Chichester: John Wiley and Sons.
Faulkner A (1985) *Nursing: A Creative Approach.* London: Baillière Tindall.

There are several monographs published by the Royal College of Nursing in the RCN Research Series, which are related to clinical nursing practice, for example:

Ashworth P (1980) *Care to Communicate: An Investigation into the Problems of Communication Between Patients and Nurses in Intensive Therapy Units.*
Atkinson F I and Sklaroff S A (1987) *Acute Hospital Wards and the Disabled Patient. A Survey of the Experiences of Patients and Nurses.*
Boore J R P (1978) *Prescription for Recovery. The Effect of Pre-operative Preparation of Surgical Patients on Post-operative Stress, Recovery and Infection.*
Coates V E (1985) *Are They Being Served? An Investigation into the Nutritional Care given by Nurses to Acute Medical Patients and the Influence of Ward Organisational Patterns on that Care.*
Fielding P (1986) *Attitudes Revisited. An Examination of Student Nurses' Attitudes Towards Old People in Hospital.*
Pearson A (1987) *Living in a Plastercast. How Nursing Can Help.*
Rodin J (1983) *Will this Hurt? Preparing Children for Hospital and Medical Procedures.*

Nursing Research

Darling V H and Rogers J (1986) *Research for Practising Nurses.* London: Macmillan.
Royal College of Nursing (1977) *Ethics Related to Research in Nursing.* London: Royal College of Nursing.

Nursing Management.

Matthews A (1982) *In Charge of the Ward*. Oxford: Blackwell Scientific Publications.

Rowden R (1984) *Managing Nursing*. London: Baillière Tindall.

Other management texts, which have been written for the busy practitioner, and are very readable, are:

Blanchard K and Lorber R (1984) *Putting the One Minute Manager to Work. A Practical Guide to Improving Performance*. Glasgow: Fontana/Collins.

Leigh A (1984) *20 Ways to Manage Better*. London: Institute of Personnel Management.

Philp T (1985) *Improving your Decision Making Skills*. London: McGraw-Hill.

Scott J and Rochester A (1984) *Effective Management Skills*:
– *What is a Manager?*
– *Managing People.*
– *Managing Money.*
– *Managing Work.*

All 4 published by Sphere/British Institute of Management.

Two rather detailed texts are:

Bowman M P (1986) *Nursing Management and Education: A Conceptual Approach to Change*. London: Croom Helm.

Hunt J W (1986) *Managing People at Work. A Manager's Guide to Behaviour in Organisations*, 2nd edn. London: McGraw-Hill.

Appendix I
Some Learning Theories

This appendix provides an introduction to some theories of learning, in order that the reader may more easily relate theory to practice. However, it is stressed that the material included here acts as a brief introduction, and the reader is strongly recommended to follow it up by reading a more detailed text such as Quinn (1988), especially chapters 1, 2, 3, 6, 7 and 16. These chapters provide a more detailed account of learning theories related to learning and teaching in the clinical area.

Categories of learning theory that will be considered are:

- *Stimulus–response theories*; also known as behaviourist, connectionist or associationist theories.
- *Cognitive theories*; also referred to as Gestalt theory or field theory.
- *Humanistic theories*; assumptions from one of these theories have already been mentioned (Rogers, 1983).
- *Other theories*; these, such as Knowles's (1984) andragogical theory of adult learning or Bandura's (1977) social learning theory, do not fit into the above but are related to learning in some situations.

No single theory accounts for all learning, and various theories overlap; however, the different theories can be grouped into four categories, and each category will be considered, with some examples of how the theories in it apply to nursing and, above all, how they can be used to enhance learning while nursing care is carried out.

STIMULUS–RESPONSE THEORIES

Possibly the best-known theorist in this group, quoted by Quinn (1988), is Pavlov, a physiologist who was interested in the digestive system. While studying salivation he recorded the unlearned physiological reflex of salivation when food was placed in a dog's mouth. He noticed that dogs salivated as they entered the laboratory, as if they had learnt to 'expect' food.

He, therefore, tested whether the dog had 'learnt' to salivate ready for food by striking a tuning fork immediately prior to giving food. After several presentations of noise with food, Pavlov presented just the noise and the dogs salivated. In other words, the dogs had learnt that the sound of the tuning fork was *associated* with the imminent arrival of food, and they therefore salivated. Pavlov regarded this salivation response to the sound as a learned rather than an innate response. He used the term *conditioning*, and the phenomenon is now known as *classical conditioning*. To recapitulate:

- **Before conditioning**: Food in the mouth (*unconditioned stimulus*) leads to salivation A (*unconditioned response*).
- **During conditioning**: Food in the mouth (*unconditioned stimulus*) plus tone (*conditioned stimulus*) leads to salivation A (*unconditioned response*).
- **After conditioning**: Tone alone (*conditioned stimulus*) leads to salivation B (*conditioned response*).

Is there a place for classical conditioning in nursing?

Exercise

Describe an instance in nursing when your actions need to be as reflexes, without having to think through a series of options.

While classical conditioning is widespread in everyday life, accounting for involuntary emotional responses such as the fear of spiders, classical conditioning has little bearing upon learning, with the possible exception of the reflex action to emergency situations, the sequence of responses to which have been learnt previously in other learning situations.

Think of an emergency situation for which you have been trained to react, perhaps cardiac arrest, arterial haemorrhage or a prolapsed umbilical cord, where spontaneous prompt action is essential and life-saving. After such an event, when asked why or how they managed to act in a particular way, people will commonly reply, 'Oh, it's instinctive', or, 'It all happened so quickly I didn't have time to think – I just got on with it'.

Your training will have taught you what action to take in such emergency situations, and you may have been taught to put those actions into motion at the sound of a particular alarm bell. The alarm bell of the monitor acts a conditioned stimulus – what you had learnt earlier becomes the conditioned response and takes over the necessary action before you have time to think!

There are one or two points about conditioning which should be mentioned.

Extinction. If the conditioned stimulus occurs on a number of occasions without the unconditioned stimulus, the conditioned response will eventually become extinct. If you leave nursing and work in a factory where a bell of similar tone to the alarm bell on the cardiac monitor sounds at the end of shift, at first you will jump and be ready for action, but gradually you will 'learn' not to respond in that way, and will merely pack up and get ready to go home.

Generalisation. If a new cardiac monitor is introduced with a slightly different tone, your response to its ringing will be the same emergency action as to the first, provided that the tones are similar.

Discrimination. One can, however, learn to discriminate between the door bell, the telephone and the alarm bell. 'Hearing dogs' for the deaf have been conditioned in this way, so that they can assist their owner to detect sounds he or she cannot hear, such as those of the baby crying.

Spontaneous Recovery. A conditioned response that has become extinct may recover without further training. If you give up nursing for a few years, your response to the alarm bell will fade, but often you are pleasantly surprised that, once you are back in a familiar situation, the swift reaction to the emergency is still there. It is also much easier to retrain than to train initially.

Another type of learning that has little place in nursing is *trial and error learning* (Quinn, 1988). Thorndike, like Pavlov, worked with animals. He confined a hungry cat in a puzzle box and put food outside the box where the cat could see it. The door to the box could be opened by a cord hanging down. The cat tried randomly scratching around to get out and, by chance, clawed the cord, opened the door and reached the food. Thorndike repeated this several times with the cat. He watched the cat's movements and noticed how long it took for the cat to escape and get the food. Gradually, the cat's actions became less random and its release was quicker, until finally, as soon as the cat was put in the box, it pulled the cord and got out to the food. Thorndike formulated the *Law of Effect*, which states that a behaviour that results in success or reward is more likely to be repeated than behaviour that does not. Another law formulated by Thorndike is the *Law of Exercise*, which states that knowledge of results must occur before behaviour can be reinforced.

Exercise

On what occasions do you think you might make use of the Law of Effect or the Law of Exercise in your work?

While there can be little place for trial and error learning in patient care, both the Law of Effect and the Law of Exercise have relevance to learning in the working area. If an activity is carried out and goes well, it is more likely to be repeated, as it is accompanied by a feeling of encouragement. For instance, if you demonstrate and teach a learner to perform a difficult manual task that she masters successfully, not only will she feel that she has achieved something, but also you will be pleased that your efforts were worthwhile, and you are likely to demonstrate to or teach other learners.

Thorndike's contribution to learning theory is the concept of *reinforcement*, which will be briefly explained in relation to the work of Skinner, who also studied conditioning as a form of learning (Quinn, 1988). Unlike Pavlov's experiments on classical conditioning, Skinner studied what has been called *operant* or *instrumental conditioning*.

Operant conditioning operates on the environment, and the learned behaviour is instrumental in controlling events. Skinner's view of operant behaviour is that the behaviour occurs spontaneously, but that reinforcement can modify it rather than it having the stimulus–response connection of Pavlov. There are a few important points to be understood in connection with reinforcement.

Positive Reinforcement. Some kind of reward follows a particular response. This increases the probability of the occurrence of the response that preceded the reward. For example, praise from a valued person following a desired behaviour will increase the likelihood of that behaviour being repeated. Thus, if the ward sister praises a staff nurse who has consoled grieving relatives with sensitivity and in a caring manner, that nurse is more likely to undertake the stressful task again with similar sensitivity.

Negative Reinforcement. If an unpleasant happening can be prevented by a particular response, the response is likely to be repeated. For example, if a student is aware that failure to complete her course work will result in termination of training, she will then work to complete the assignment on time, to avoid the unpleasant situation of being discharged from the course. Therefore, negative reinforcement *increases* the occurrence of the response which precedes it.

Punishment. Punishment differs from negative reinforcement in that the unpleasant happening occurs after the response. If a nurse makes an error in drug administration she is likely to be disciplined. Punishment *decreases* the probability of occurrence of the response which precedes it.

Omission of Reinforcement. If there is no reinforcement after a response, the response is likely to diminish. Skinner described various *schedules of reinforcement*, when the rate of reinforcement is varied in different ways, which reduce the likelihood of omission of a response.

Shaping. Shaping implies the incorporation of new behaviours into the repertoire of an individual's behaviour. This may be used to assist mentally handicapped individuals in learning social skills or even basic skills, such as feeding and dressing. Reinforcement is given when behaviour that approximates to what is required occurs. As the responses move nearer to the desired activity they are rewarded, thus shaping the behaviour.

Exercise

List the common stimulus–response theories and give alongside each one an example from your work.

COGNITIVE THEORIES

Cognition is a term given to the mental processes such as thinking, problem-solving, remembering and perceiving.

Gestalt Psychology and Insight Learning

This work began as a study of perception; the Gestalt view is that people see things as wholes. ('Gestalt' is a German word meaning pattern or configuration.) The patterns, or Gestalten, tend to stand out distinctly from the background against which they are seen. The Gestalt psychologists formulated laws of perception that govern whether or not a stimulus is seen as a figure.

Law of Similarity

Things that are similar to one another tend to be grouped together, e.g.:

```
. + . + . +
. + . + . +
. + . + . +
. + . + . +
```

tends to be seen as alternating columns of . and +, rather than as a square with 24 symbols.

Law of Proximity

Stimuli or things which are close together tend to be grouped together, e.g.:

tends to be seen as two pairs of horizontal lines, rather than as four separate lines.

These two 'laws' also help when considering memory, since like or similar pieces of information may be grouped together and learnt as a whole, or at least in chunks, thus taking up less memory space. Think about remembering telephone numbers. It is much easier to remember them in groups of numbers, i.e. the area code followed by the subscriber's number, rather than as a string of seven or eight numbers; for example, 745 3452 is easier to recall than 7453452. Therefore, when in the clinical situation think about how to present information, like with like, so that the listener does not have to perform mental gymnastics in order to keep up with the flow.

Law of Closure

Incomplete lines that enclose a space are more inclined to form a Gestalt or whole and, therefore, to stand out against a background. This law also has implications for the clinical area, in that what we 'see' may not be so; this can be beneficial, but may also be misleading. Think of instances when a judgment is based mainly on what is seen, such as the cyanosis of a patient or the hyperactivity of a child!

Kurt Koffka considered that these laws of perception could be applied to learning and used in teaching. The learning described in Gestalt psychology is called *insightful learning* (Quinn, 1988). Possibly the best remembered is the work of Kohler, which he carried out with a chimpanzee, who was kept in a cage with some bananas suspended above it, just out of his reach. In the cage were some boxes scattered around. The chimpanzee could not reach the bananas by standing on one of the boxes, but after various attempts, the animal sat quietly for a time, then sudenly piled the boxes one on top of the other and retrieved the bananas. Kohler interpreted the behaviour of the chimpanzee as that of gaining insight into the problem by seeing the boxes and the banana in a new relationship, which became meaningful, and he was thus able to solve the problem. To relate the laws of perception to the learning, both the boxes and the bananas were in the animal's visual field at the same time (Law of Proximity). The Law of Closure is demonstrated by the relationship of the boxes being seen as a means of reaching the bananas. The sudden insight of how to solve a problem is termed the 'aha' *phenomenon.*

You may well have experienced a similar feeling when the solution to a problem that had been bothering you suddenly came to mind, or you may have seen it occur to someone else. For example, suppose one is doing a drug round with a student nurse, who has difficulty in calculating the number of tablets to be given when the prescription is written as 0.5 g and the tablets in the bottle are of 250 mg. Once she knows that there are 1 000 mg in a gram and that 0.5 is half, she should be able to see quickly that half of 1000 is 500, and that two 250 mg tablets will make 500 mg. Until she has an understanding of the relationship of milligrams to grams, all is a mystery; once given the necessary information, not only does she suddenly see the relationship, but also she will be able to work out other doses that may have been puzzling her.

More recently Ausubel (1978) has used a cognitive approach to learning, *assimilation theory*, which is what it sounds like – new information is incorporated into existing knowledge. According to Ausubel's theory, most meaningful cognitive learning occurs as a result of interaction between new information and the cognitive structures that the learner already possesses. He sees what the learner already knows as the most important factor in influencing further learning. Ausubel suggests that it may be necessary to use an advance organiser, in the form of introductory material that is taught to the student ahead of the main body of information. The advance organiser provides a specific anchoring structure upon which the learner can build. The advance organiser acts as a bridge between what the student already knows and the new information. When trying to help a nurse to understand a disease process, find out first of all if she understands the healthy/normal process. It will be diffcult to help her to understand what is wrong with a patient if she has no clear idea of what a fit person is like.

Information-Processing Approach

There are various information-processing theories, but, basically, these propose a model to explain how information in the environment is attended to selectively, then passed to the short-term memory and on to the long-term memory, where it is stored. Sensory memory registers incoming stimuli for between 1 and 5 seconds, an example being the persistence of a spot of light in the dark after the light has been switched off. Short-term memory has a storage capacity of seven 'chunks' of information. The 'chunk' or 'bit' of information applies to a unit of information, which may be a single letter or a whole phrase, so long as the phrase is processed as one chunk; it is, therefore, possible to increase the amount held in the short-term memory by increasing the information in each chunk. There appears to be no such limit in the long-term memory. Rehearsing short-term memory, called *maintenance rehearsal*, consists of repeatedly going over the information held in the short-term memory, thus keeping it there. The elaborative memory processes material in the long-term memory. There are various theories of how information is stored in long-term memory. Some of the theories refer to *schema*, which make up the building blocks of the human information processing system. One definition of a schema was given by Anderson in 1980:

'large, complex units of knowledge that organise much of what we know about general categories of objects, classes of events and types of people'.

In long-term memory the information is classified; it can then be retrieved and affect a particular response or behaviour. For example, although there is much activity and noise in a busy ward or department, an experienced nurse will be alerted by hearing significant sounds that penetrate the general background clatter, such as the stertorous breathing of a comatose patient who needs immediate attention. She will straight away investigate and take the necessary remedial action. The nurse's selective attention detected the distressed breathing, the sound of which was coded and passed through her short-term memory to the long-term meomory, where classification of the stimulus resulted in identification of that sound as a danger signal needing an urgent response. Previous experience had taught her that this kind of sound could indicate a life-threatening situation, and thus the initiation of the response to clear the airway occurred.

There has been much research demonstrating that only a limited amount of information, seven 'chunks' or 'bits', can be processed at one time (Miller, 1956). This is important when one tries to impart information, perhaps on introducing a new member to the work area. It should always be remembered that there is a limit to what an individual can take in, even without the inhibitory effect of anxiety. Remember Gestalt psychology and the Laws of Similarity and Proximity, and group similar incidents or facts together.

HUMANISTIC THEORIES OF LEARNING

Humanistic theories are exactly the opposite of the stimulus–response theories considered earlier. Whereas stimulus–response theories look at the resultant behaviour, humanistic theories study the whole person – thoughts, feelings and experiences. Humanistic theories are concerned with human growth, individual fulfilment and self-actualisation. The emphasis of the theories is on teacher–student relationship and the learning climate. Maslow (1970) sees education as helping the person to make the best of himself. Surely, this is the crucial aim for all health-care workers – to give the best care of which they are capable. The motivation comes from within the person as the desire to develop and grow. Maslow sees self-actualisation as the ultimate aim of learning.

Another theorist who looks at the person as a whole is Rogers (1983). His student-centred approach to education states that we can only enable or facilitate people to learn, and that they will only learn what they see as being important for their needs. Rogers also emphasises the importance of a learning environment that is free from threat. Much research has been focused in this area of nurse learning in the UK, and has been discussed in more detail in Chapter 2.

OTHER THEORIES RELATED TO LEARNING

Knowles's Andragogical Theory

Andragogy is the art and science of teaching adults. Knowles (1984) describes several assumptions, which show andragogy to be different from pedagogy, the teaching usually related to children, upon which, until recently, much educational practice was based. It is worth taking a brief look at the assumptions, as they relate well to health-care workers and their patients and clients.

The Need to Know

Adults need to know why they have to learn something before they undertake to learn it. In nursing, it is often clear why something has to be learnt, but there are times when a difficult task has to be mastered despite the fact that the use of the knowledge or skill is not immediately apparent. Putting the task into the context of why it is to be learnt, or how it might affect patient care, can help learners to cope with the task. For example, it is important that certain actions and procedures be followed precisely at the time of a cardiac arrest, while at other times, care can be modified to meet the individual's needs.

The Learners' Self-Concept

Adults have a self-concept of being responsible for their own decisions and their own lives, and, therefore, expect to be treated by others as if they are capable of self-direction. Nurse learners have been heard to complain about the way they are treated – as being unable to think for themselves as learners, yet, at the same time, being treated as working adults, able to care for other individuals. Nurse training was based on a pedagogical model developed from schooling, and ill prepared learner nurses for the tasks ahead (Gott, 1984). It is hoped that the introduction of Project 2000 in the UK will enable a thorough review of teaching practice to take place.

The Role of the Learner's Experience

Adults come into an educational activity with a vast variety of experiences. These experiences can be a rich source on which to build, but some may have unwanted affects if they result in negative attitudes towards a topic, or in biases which may prohibit learning. For example, if a student nurse has a beloved grandparent who is kind, clean and of sound mind, she may have positive attitudes towards care of the elderly. If, however, the student has had to spend her Saturday afternoons minding a querulous grandparent rather than being out with her friends, she may then have rather negative attitudes towards care of the elderly.

Readiness to Learn

Adults become ready to learn what they need to know in order to function more efficiently. Therefore, a woman pregnant for the first time will eagerly learn about parentcraft and her own health routines, in order to give birth to a healthy baby. Sometimes a person may need help to 'open up' so that he or she can acknowledge a need to learn. This is more likely to occur if there is a supportive environment. Change and anxiety inhibit the readiness to learn; the NHS has suffered from much change, with resultant anxiety.

Orientation to Learning

Adults learn more effectively when new knowledge, understanding, skills, values and attitudes are presented in the context of applications to real life situations. Take the example of neurological observations and recordings: these can be quite complex for the inexperienced nurse, but if she understands the significance of pupil size and reaction to the condition of the child with head injuries, she will be more likely to remember what she has been taught and why it is necessary to carry out the observations (the importance of relating theory to practice was discussed in Chapter 2).

Motivation

Adults will respond to external motivators, like a better job or a higher salary, but more potent are the internal motivators such as self-esteem and quality of life.

It can be seen from the brief mention of three of the humanistic theories of learning that there is a common theme running through them, namely, the need of the adult learner for enhancement of self-respect or self-esteem through learning.

Bandura's Social Learning Theory

In 1977, Bandura proposed that learning is a two-way interaction between the individual and the environment. According to his social learning theory, an individual has no patterns of behaviour other than reflexes, and learns all behaviour by observing other people. The importance of learning by observation cannot be dismissed in the context of learning in the work-place. The importance of the ward sister as role model for her nursing staff has been demonstrated in several studies (see Chapter 2).

Gagne (1985) says:

> 'One of the most dependable sets of events that has been found to produce changes in attitudes is the phenomenon of human modelling.'

In role modelling, a person who is respected or admired exhibits certain behaviours. When these behaviours are then observed by someone else, they are taken to indicate desirable behaviours or attitudes. For example, when in 1980 Pembrey asked the ward sisters participating in her research study how they had learnt how to be a sister, several said that they had worked with a good sister during their training or when they were a staff nurse, and had tried to follow her example. If a sister who is respected and admired demonstrates an unhurried, caring attitude towards patients' relatives, the nurses will identify those behaviours and attitudes as the 'correct' way to behave, and will then be likely to copy them and emulate the sister. This is good when the role model demonstrates desired attitudes or behaviours; however, nurses may be role models for their patients, and nurses who are seen to be smoking in the dining room, for example, will not demonstrate a health-conscious attitude or be a desirable role model.

The final point to be discussed is not really a theory but a drawing together of many factors which influence learning.

Gagne's Conditions of Learning. The main idea in Gagne's system is that all human learning can be classified into five varieties of capability, and these capabilities cover all types of learning. Once the learning outcomes have been identified, the conditions which govern learning and remembering can be accounted for.

Having briefly looked at some of the theories of learning, and seen that some theories are more applicable to certain types of learning than others, it is hoped that an insight into the variety of ways in which theory can help the promotion of learning in the work-place has been provided. Selecting the most appropriate method of encouraging learning is likely to pay dividends, as the individual is likely to learn more quickly, thereby saving time and energy. But above all, in the context of patient care, the more quickly the nurse learns, the better it is for the patient.

References

Anderson J (1980) *Cognitive Psychology and its Implications.* San Francisco: W H Freeman.

Ausubel D (1978) *Educational Psychology: A Cognitive View.* New York: Holt, Rinehart and Winston.

Bandura A (1977) *Social Learning Theory.* New Jersey: Prentice Hall.

Gagne R M (1985) *The Conditions of Learning and the Theory of Instruction.* New York: Holt, Rinehart and Winston.

Gott M (1984) *Learning Nursing. A Study of the Effectiveness and Relevance of Teaching Provided During Student Nurse Introductory Course.* RCN Research Series. London: Royal College of Nursing.

Knowles M (1984) *The Adult Learner: A Neglected Species.* Houston: Gulf Publishing Co.

Maslow A H (1970) *Motivation and Personality.* New York: Harper and Row.

Miller G A (1956) The magical number seven plus or minus two: some limits on our capacity for processing information. *Psychological Review,* **63**: 81–99.

Pembrey S (1980) *The Ward Sister – Key to Nursing. A Study of the Organisation of Individualised Nursing.* RCN Research Series. London: Royal College of Nursing.

Quinn F M (1988) *The Principles and Practice of Nurse Education.* London: Croom Helm.

Rogers C R (1983) *Freedom to Learn in the Eighties.* Columbus, Ohio: Charles E Merrill.

Appendix II
Code of Professional Conduct for the Nurse, Midwife and Health Visitor

Published by the United Kingdom Council for Nursing, Midwifery and Health Visiting, 2nd edn., 1984.

Each registered nurse, midwife and health visitor shall act, at all times, in such a manner as to justify public trust and confidence, to uphold and enhance the good standing and reputation of the profession, to serve the interests of society, and above all to safeguard the interests of individual patients and clients.

Each registered nurse, midwife and health visitor is accountable for his or her practice, and, in the exercise of professional accountability shall:

1. Act always in such a way as to promote and safeguard the well being and interests of patients/clients.
2. Ensure that no action or omission on his/her part or within his/her sphere of influence is detrimental to the condition or safety of patients/clients.
3. Take every reasonable opportunity to maintain and improve professional knowledge and competence.
4. Acknowledge any limitations of competence and refuse in such cases to accept delegated functions without first having received instruction in regard to those functions and having been assessed as competent.
5. Work in a collaborative and co-operative manner with other health care professionals and recognise and respect their particular contributions within the health care team.
6. Take account of the customs, values and spiritual beliefs of patients/clients.
7. Make known to an appropriate person or authority any conscientious objection which may be relevant to professional practice.
8. Avoid any abuse of the privileged relationship which exists with patients/clients and of the privileged access allowed to their property, residence or workplace.

126

9. Respect confidential information obtained in the course of professional practice and refrain from disclosing such information without the consent of the patient/client, or a person entitled to act on his/her behalf, expect where disclosure is required by law or by the order of a court or is necessary in the public interest.
10. Have regard to the environment of care and its physical, psychological and social effects on patients/clients, and also to the adequacy of resources, and make known to appropriate persons or authorities any circumstances which could place patients/clients in jeopardy or which militate against safe standards of practice.
11. Have regard to the workload of and the pressures on professional colleagues and subordinates and take appropriate action if these are seen to be such as to constitute abuse of the individual practitioner and/or to jeopardise safe standards of practice.
12. In the context of the individual's own knowledge, experience, and sphere of authority, assist peers and subordinates to develop professional competence in accordance with their needs.
12. Refuse to accept any gift, favour or hospitality which might be interpreted as seeking to exert undue influence to obtain preferential consideration.
14. Avoid the use of professional qualifications in the promotion of commercial products in order not to compromise the independence of professional judgement on which patients/clients rely.

Notice to all Registered Nurses, Midwives and Health Visitors

This Code of Professional Conduct is issued by the United Kingdom Central Council for Nursing, Midwifery and Health Visiting.

It is issued for the guidance and advice of all registered nurses, midwives and health visitors.

Further explanatory notes, discussion papers or comments on specific points in the Code of Professional Conduct may be issued by the Council from time to time.

The Code will be subject to periodic review by the Council.

The Council expects members of the profession to recognise it as their responsibility (as well as the Council's) to re-appraise the relevance of the Code to the professional and social context in which they practice.

The Council will welcome suggestions and comments for consideration in its periodic review of the Code of Professional Conduct.

(Reproduced by kind permission of UKCC)

Appendix III
Code for Nurses with Interpretive Statements

Published in 1985 by the American Nurses' Association, 2420 Pershing Road, Kansas City, Missouri. (Only p.1 is reproduced.)

1. The nurse provides services with respect for human dignity and the uniqueness of the client, unrestricted by considerations of social or economic status, personal attributes, or the nature of health problems.
2. The nurse safeguards the client's right to privacy by judiciously protecting information of a confidential nature.
3. The nurse acts to safeguard the client and the public when health care and safety are affected by the incompetent, unethical, or illegal practice of any person.
4. The nurse assumes responsibility and accountability for individual nursing judgments and actions.
5. The nurse maintains competence in nursing.
6. The nurse exercises informed judgment and uses individual competence and qualifications as criteria in seeking consultation, accepting responsibilities, and delegating nursing activities to others.
7. The nurse participates in activities that contribute to the ongoing developments of the profession's body of knowledge.
8. The nurse participates in the profession's efforts to implement and improve standards of nursing.
9. The nurse participates in the profession's efforts to establish and maintain conditions of employment conducive to high quality nursing care.
10. The nurse participates in the profession's effort to protect the public from misinformation and misrepresentation and to maintain the integrity of nursing.
11. The nurse collaborates with members of the health professions and other citizens in promoting community and national efforts to meet the health needs of the public.

(Reproduced by kind permission of the American Nurses' Association)

Index